Full text of articles available at:
http://www.unescap.org/pop/journal/index.htm

ASIA-PACIFIC POPULATION JOURNAL

June 2003

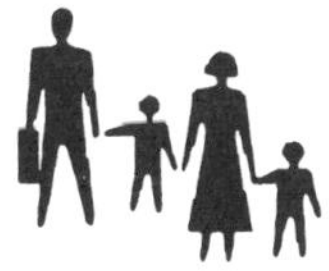

CO[NTENTS]

Abstra[cts]	2
Article[s]	

UNESCAP works towards reducing poverty and managing globalization

Page

Evolution of Population Concerns: Reflections from the Asian and Pacific Population Conferences

5

The purposes, themes, organization, agenda items and debates of the five decennial Asian and Pacific Population Conferences are described by the author, who participated in all five Conferences. The technical and financial support given by the United Nations and its specialized agencies as well as the Commission secretariat to the countries of Asia and the Pacific in undertaking their population and development programmes is also depicted. From a simple consideration of the demographic situation in 1963, the succeeding Conferences manifested the growing sophistication of the region in the choice of issues to be considered and in the debates and actions taken by the Governments in confronting those issues.

The Fifth Asian and Pacific Population Conference: Towards a Repositioning of Population in the Global Development Agenda?

21

Since the Bali Conference 10 years earlier, by the time of the Fifth Asian and Pacific Population Conference at Bangkok in December 2002, the Asian and Pacific region had become more diverse demographically, though with a clear shift towards lower fertility and mortality levels. Economically, the region had grown impressively, albeit with considerable variation. In Bangkok, there was less sense of the urgency of lowering fertility rates, and indeed in some countries the issue had become one of needing to raise these rates. These countries and areas held firm to the reproductive health emphases of the Cairo Programme of Action, despite the concerns of the United States of America delegation that the language of the Programme of Action tended to promote abortion and adolescent sexual activity. The Plan of Action on Population and Poverty adopted by consensus at the conclusion of the Conference is a carefully worded document, reflecting current consensus about principles and broad directions for action in the areas of population and development. Though the population issue as conventionally understood no longer appears an urgent concern, there is a need to recognize that population and development issues are just as important for countries with low fertility as they are for countries with high fertility. Moreover, there are important population dimensions of the issues that are currently given the greatest prominence, including poverty and environmental sustainability.

Knowledge of Sexual Health Issues among Unmarried Young People in Nepal   33

Evidence from other country settings shows that sex education delivered in school can make a positive contribution to children and young people's knowledge and personal and social development, helping to prevent negative health outcomes such as unintended pregnancies and sexually transmitted infections. Using data collected from a survey of over 1,000 students from six secondary schools in Nepal, this paper explores young people's knowledge of sexual health issues and sources of information.

The data show that detailed knowledge regarding many sexual health issues is low among both young men and women, although exposure to visual media messages and access to informative sources of literature can have a positive impact. Schools appear to play an important role in informing young people about sexual health matters; however, further curriculum and teacher training material development is required with a shift away from superficial biological coverage towards a more inclusive programme.

Reproductive Health including Family Planning   55

This paper reviews the role of family planning in reproductive health in the Asian and Pacific region since the International Conference on Population and Development (ICPD) in 1994. It also identifies areas in reproductive health that should be priorities over the next decade. The Asian and Pacific region has made impressive advances in implementing the recommendations of ICPD. Even though concern has been expressed that an emphasis on reproductive health would diminish the role of family planning, the experience in the region over the last decade has been that the integration of family planning into expanded reproductive health programmes that provide women and men with choice in planning their reproductive lives did not lead to reversals in fertility decline. There remain several areas where recommendations from the Programme of Action have faced difficulties in implementation and where more attention is required. The development of adolescent reproductive health programmes has been hampered by the widespread belief that unmarried adolescents should not be exposed to information and/or services related to reproductive health. Entrenched systems that support gender inequality restrict reproductive choices available to women. Additional attention also needs to be placed on the interrelationships between sexual and reproductive health.

Evolution of Population Concerns: Reflections from the Asian and Pacific Population Conferences

*It is imperative that the population community
sustain its efforts to keep the population perspective
in the forefront of issues such as globalization, environment
and sustainable development*

By Mercedes B. Concepcion*

The United Nations Seminar on Population in Asia and the Far East, held at Bandung, Indonesia, in 1955, focused attention on increasing population trends within the region covered by the Economic Commission for Asia and the Far East (ECAFE). The Seminar realized that the current rising population growth rates largely negated or probably even retarded the effects of national socio-economic

---

* Commissioner, Philippines Commission on Population. Dr. Concepcion has attended all the Population Conferences starting from the First Asian Population Conference, held at New Delhi in 1963.

programmes that provided an environment conducive to lowering birth rates. Interest in the region's population gains was further stimulated by the establishment of the Demographic Training and Research Centre at Bombay, India, jointly operated by the United Nations and the Government of India. At the Centre's inaugural conference it was suggested that the United Nations convene a regional conference on population. That proposal was taken up by the Commission in its resolution 28 (XV) of 13 March 1959 requesting the secretariat to organize an Asian population conference where experts could examine the major problems of planning for economic and social development arising from current and prospective trends in population growth, composition and geographic distribution. Consequently, in 1963, the First Asian Population Conference (APC) was held at New Delhi, with the Government of India providing host facilities. APC was established as a statutory organ of the Commission to be convened every 10 years to consider all aspects of population questions and, of their impact on economic and social development as mandated in Commission resolution 74 (XXIII) of 17 April 1967.

The Second APC, hosted by the Government of Japan, was held at Tokyo in November 1972. In 1974, the name of ECAFE was changed to Economic and Social Commission for Asia and the Pacific (ESCAP). Five years later, in line with its enlarged scope, the Commission decided that APC should thereafter be referred to as the Asian and Pacific Population Conference (APPC). The Third and Fourth APPCs were convened at Colombo in September 1982 and at Bali, Indonesia, in August 1992, respectively. The most recent APPC was held at Bangkok in December 2002. Today, half a year after the Fifth APPC, it seems appropriate to reflect on the evolution of issues and opinions since the 1963 Conference.

The following paragraphs will describe the development of the Conferences in terms of participation, organization and especially the debate on emerging issues in response to the changing demographic scene. The population growth pattern and the general locale that prompted the discussions during the first and subsequent Conferences will be set forth. The role of the United Nations, especially ESCAP, in placing population issues on the agendas of Governments across the Asian and Pacific region will also be portrayed.

Organization

Purpose

The First APC provided a forum where experts examined the major problems of planning for economic and social development arising from present and prospective trends in population growth, composition and distribution. During the Second APC, participants arrived at a better understanding of the central role of population in achieving development goals. Governments in the region were assisted in ascertaining and applying the most effective means of influencing population trends and patterns in order to hasten the attainment of the Second United Nations Development Decade goals. A further understanding of the two-way interrelationships between population and development and the need to consider relevant factors fully in the formulation and implementation of policies and programmes to achieve overall national development goals were the aims of the Third APPC. The Fourth APPC enabled Governments in the region to understand clearly the strategic value of formulating multidisciplinary policies and programmes, to realize the need to integrate research and evaluation into programme planning and implementation and to appreciate the role of population data and information in policy formulation and programme implementation. Progress made in implementing the recommendations contained in the Bali Declaration, the Programme of Action of the International Conference on Population and Development (ICPD), the five-year reviews and appraisals of the Bali Declaration and the ICPD Programme of Action, the Platform for Action of the Fourth World Conference on Women and the Millennium Declaration adopted at the United Nations Millennium Summit was reviewed during the Fifth APPC.

Participation

Participation in the Conferences more than doubled from some 20 members and associate members in the ECAFE region in 1963 to 42 ESCAP members and associate members in 2002. Selected non-governmental organizations (NGOs) and foundations were invited to attend the First APC. In attendance were the trainees and staff of the Bombay Demographic Training and Research Centre.

In addition to the 21 ECAFE members and associate members, United Nations bodies, United Nations specialized agencies and NGOs, 38 experts in demography and related disciplines were appointed as resource persons to assist in the Second APC, held in 1972. A decade later, 32 members and associate members of the Commission took part in the Third APPC together with representatives of United Nations bodies, intergovernmental organizations, NGOs and observers from various organizations in the region. In Bali, the Fourth APPC changed in format with two different segments: senior officials from 36 members and associate members of ESCAP gathering first for six days, followed by a two-day meeting of ministers from 40 members and associate members of the region. Forty-two members and associate members sent their senior officials to the Fifth APPC while 26 ministers from 23 countries were present during the ministerial meeting. A large number of representatives from United Nations Headquarters, United Nations bodies, United Nations specialized agencies as well as intergovernmental organizations and NGOs registered for these last two Conferences.

Opening addresses

Heads of State have usually inaugurated the Conference. In his opening address, Prime Minister Jawaharlal Nehru stated that the New Delhi Conference was the first to deal with subjects that were highly important to the world at large and to Asia in particular. The ECAFE countries and areas faced a race between the growth rates of the economy and that of population, he explained, hoping that the Conference would initiate a combined approach to common problems in the region with assistance from non-Asian countries.

Inaugurating the Second APC, the Japanese Vice-Prime Minister Takeo Miki stressed that Asia was the focal point of the world population problem and anticipated that the 1970s would be for Asia an age of action closely tied to policy. He counted upon the Second APC to provide momentum for the attainment of the Second United Nations Development Decade objectives.

The President of Sri Lanka, J.R. Jayewardene, observed in front of the representatives gathered for the Third APPC that Asian and Pacific countries experienced similar demographic problems where the solution applied in one situation could be adapted in another with modifications to suit local social, political, cultural and economic needs. He perceived great scope for regional cooperation in the population field among ESCAP countries and areas. The Prime Minister of Sri Lanka, R. Premadasa, urged the Third APPC to seriously consider adopting a regional population plan of action.

The Minister of State for Population and Environment of Indonesia, Emil Salim, speaking to the senior officials assembled at Bali for the Fourth APPC, stressed that the adoption of a participatory approach to cover the broadest possible range of issues would be most appropriate for reconciling population concerns, environmental factors and development objectives. In inaugurating the Meeting of Ministers, President Soeharto of Indonesia remarked that development not merely dealt with economic growth and related issues, rather it concerned people and whether they could live decently and prosperously. Future generations in the region might have a better quality of life if the resolutions and recommendations of the Fourth APPC were implemented.

Sudarat Keyuraphan, Minister of Public Health of Thailand, in her address to the Senior Officials Meeting at Bangkok, observed that the strategies and approaches introduced in earlier APPCs and ICPD by providing specific goals and a focused framework within a specific time frame would help to reduce poverty and improve the people's quality of life. The best practices or lessons learned from neighbouring countries could provide valuable models for this purpose and strengthen partnership through South-South cooperation. Inaugurating the Meeting of Ministers, Thaksin Shinawatra, Prime Minister of Thailand, stated that the recommendations emerging from the discussions during the Senior Officials Meeting provided the ministers with important guidelines for interventions and policies to promote informed choice, create opportunities, reduce poverty and improve the welfare and quality of life of people in the region.

The Secretary-General of the United Nations, the Executive Secretary of the Commission and the Executive Director of the United Nations Population Fund (UNFPA) also gave opening statements or had their messages read before the Delegations. To draw attention to the 1974 United Nations World Population Conference (WPC), Antonio Carrillo-Flores, WPC Secretary-General, stated that the Second APC paved the way for the 1974 WPC. In the same manner, speaking to the senior officials assembled in Bali in 1992, the Secretary-General of the 1994 ICPD elaborated on the policy agenda for the future, observing that the APPCs had come to symbolize leadership in the population and development field.

Agenda

The agendas of the five Conferences varied from simple consideration of the regional demographic situation and the economic and social implications of prospective population trends in 1963 to issues related to the themes adopted at the Conferences that followed. Recurring topics for the first four Conferences were the demographic situation and future outlook, research and training and information dissemination. The First APC participants unanimously adopted a resolution inviting Commission members to adopt a positive population policy related to their individual needs, keeping in mind the Conference recommendations relating to national population policies when formulating and executing their general socio-economic development policies and plans.

Family planning programmes and the ecological implications of rural and urban change were two new topics introduced at the Second APC. Held during the Second United Nations Development Decade, the Conference adopted a Declaration of Population Strategy for Development containing recommendations ranging from labour utilization to land reform, from pollution to planning mechanisms and from contraception to construction.

Under the theme "An integrated approach to population and related developmental issues", representatives at the Third APPC reviewed the progress made by members in implementing the recommendations of the World Population Plan of Action approved at Bucharest in 1974 and considered actions to be taken in the future. The formulation and implementation of integrated population and development policies and urbanization and the growth of cities were added to the agenda along with the evaluation of integrated family planning/family welfare/family health programme schemes and strategies. With the Commission enlarged to embrace the Pacific countries and areas, the population problems of small island States gained prominence. In response to the urging of the Prime Minister of Sri Lanka, a regional population plan of action, the Asia-Pacific Call for Action on Population and Development, was adopted by the delegations during the plenary session.

The theme chosen for the Fourth APPC was "Population and sustainable development: goals and strategies into the twenty-first century". The agenda included a discussion of the socio-economic implications of population ageing as well as human resources development and poverty alleviation issues. After examining the population situation and outlook and noting the substantial progress achieved by the region's countries in responding to the Asia-Pacific Call for Action on Population and Development adopted at the previous APPC, the meeting of ministers adopted the Bali Declaration on Population and Sustainable Development.

The theme of the Fifth APPC, "Population and poverty in Asia and the Pacific", emphasized the need to re-evaluate the links between population and development and to crystallize and revitalize the thinking on the links between population and poverty in the light of the United Nations Millennium Declaration adopted in 2000. To highlight the theme, the first agenda item taken up was population and poverty in Asia and the Pacific. Adolescent reproductive health, HIV/AIDS and poverty, gender equality and development, behavioural change communication and advocacy as tools for population and development and poverty reduction were new topics covered in the Bangkok agenda. The senior officials strongly reaffirmed their commitment to the ICPD Programme of Action, which continued to serve as their guide in undertaking their reproductive health programmes. Future activities to advance the Bali and ICPD agendas to reflect realistically the needs of the region's countries and their expectations from international partners towards meeting those needs are embodied in the Fifth Asian and Pacific Population Conference Plan of Action on Population and Poverty adopted by the meeting of ministers after a vote.

The debates

Knowledge and understanding of the demographic situation and population problems of most countries in the region were still rudimentary at the time of the First APC despite progress made since the 1955 Bandung Seminar. In 1963, only a few Governments recognized the implications of high population growth rates. Only five administrations in the region had official population policies. The region's population totalled about 1.7 billion. Recognizing the role of demographic factors in economic and social development, the representatives stressed that moderation of population growth was a matter of great urgency and family size limitation should be accorded the highest possible priority in development programmes. Industrialization, land reform and other programmes were recognized to have accelerated socio-economic development. The Conference agreed that rapid population growth in many of the region's less developed countries was impeding socio-economic progress and threatening the success of efforts to reach satisfactory levels of living within a tolerable length of time. The Conference called on the United Nations and its specialized agencies to expand the scope of their technical assistance. The Commission was requested to: (a) strengthen its regional advisory services in the demographic field; (b) increase opportunities for qualified students from countries in the region to obtain fellowships for advanced studies in demography and related fields; (c) strengthen its secretariat assigned to work on population matters so as to enable it to render effective services to government agencies and institutions working in this field; (d) compile and analyse statistical data and other information on the demography of countries in the region, and prepare reports for publication on various aspects of the demographic situation and prospects in the region and the interrelation of population trends with social and economic development; and (e) arrange for fundamental research on population questions to be carried out by universities and research institutions within the region in coordination with the Asian Institute for Economic Development and Planning and other regional demographic training and research facilities.

In 1972, the region's population had risen to 2.1 billion. Fifteen member countries had official population policies and another 10 were actively supporting family planning programmes. Against this backdrop, the Second APC considered the need to formulate population policies and programmes as integral parts of the social and economic development process and recognized the two-way relationship of population with socio-economic development. The delegations stressed that reducing infant and maternal mortality, achieving full and productive employment, abating excessive migration flows to the larger cities and improving the status of women ensured a more equitable distribution of opportunity and income. Governments seeking to fufil the ideals of their people and their national goals through population policies and programmes should: (a) provide information, education and services for all their citizens as early as possible; (b) encourage smaller families in rural and urban areas through intensive information, education and communication efforts together with the enactment of appropriate socio-economic measures; (c) consider establishing population commissions or other bodies having multidisciplinary and multidepartmental representation to assess the current status and future needs in the population and family planning fields; (d) ensure coordination among various agencies at all levels in order to expedite action on integrated development policies and plans; (e) provide essential training facilities to improve management and planning skills, and promote comprehensive and innovative population policies to increase population and family planning programme administrative capabilities; (f) encourage the development of new communication tools and utilization of existing ones so that knowledge might be shared at all levels of society; and (g) include provisions in population policy and programmes to ensure that all pertinent information reached policy makers, opinion leaders and socio-economic planners.

With a population exceeding 2.5 billion in 1982, the ESCAP region witnessed significant declines in fertility and mortality. However, population growth rates were higher than desired in 16 countries while 10 still had life expectancies of 50 years or under. Sixteen countries had fertility reduction policies and an even greater number supported family planning programmes. At the Third APPC, participants pointed out that most ESCAP countries and areas recognized the integrated approach. However, that approach had included maternal and child health since the early 1970s and more recently other programmes such as those related to the status of women had been added. While population programme managers were willing to involve other development sectors, corresponding responses had not always been forthcoming from the other sectors. The problem centred on how to design a coordinated approach to population and development policies so as to obtain the support of other sectors. The slow progress of integration was due both to the limited knowledge base relating to diverse population processes and to a likelihood that planning structures and approaches had become rigid, thus precluding the needs of population planning being taken into account. Population programmes had to be accorded an appropriate place in a Government's political and administrative structure. High-level population units had to be established within development planning organizations responsible for integrating population policies and programmes with related social and economic development policies and programmes. The concept of integration and the policies relating to integration of family planning services with other programmes had also to consider the programme recipients' viewpoint. An effective monitoring system needed to be established to undertake systematic and periodic evaluation of integrated population policies and programmes. Programmes that resulted in diminishing demand for large families should be given priority with a view to creating a socio-economic environment conducive to reducing the population growth rate.

Although considerable progress has been made in the matter of implementing population programmes, a wide gap exists between current fertility and mortality levels and fertility and mortality goals. For the first time, the 1982 APPC included population goals in its Asia-Pacific Call for Action. Existing targets and goals for reducing birth and death rates must be reviewed and modified to attain low levels as early as possible and attain a replacement level of fertility by the year 2000. Towards that end, the necessary information, education and a variety of means to practice family planning freely, effectively and in accordance with their cultural values and religious beliefs should be available and accessible to all couples and individuals. Family planning services should be strengthened though the involvement of local population and local institutions in planning, funding and implementing family planning information and services. Programme personnel should be reoriented to make family planning programmes more sensitive and responsive to local values and individual needs.

The small island countries and areas of the ESCAP region, because of their size, are economically, socially, environmentally and even demographically vulnerable. Thus, particular attention is required to protect their demographic and cultural viability. This is especially true for those countries subject to emigration. Hence, small island countries and areas, particularly those subject to emigration, were enjoined to formulate social, economic and population policies that would maintain their demographic and cultural viability.

A revolution in thinking about population issues had occurred in the ESCAP region since 1963. Many Governments had launched ambitious programmes with the result that the average annual population growth rate for Asia and the Pacific was just over 1.7 per cent in 1990 with a population numbering around 3.3 billion. The delegations to the Fourth APPC saw that high population growth and density in many countries had caused various environmental and related problems: continuing depletion and degradation of vital natural resources, the persistence of poverty among the rural population and a growing rural-urban income gap, increasing and competing demands for land, water and forests by the non-agricultural sectors and growing urban population, and deteriorating environmental quality owing to unregulated industrial and urban growth. To overcome those problems, the policies and strategies formulated should include development of environmentally friendly technology, reforestation, improvement of air and water quality, waste recycling and the phasing-out of environmentally harmful technology, improving environmental organization, administration and management, as well as appropriate laws and effective law enforcement.

The Bali Conference was concerned that the growing threat to the environment and urban infrastructure posed by rural-urban migration and by the high rate of natural increase in the urban population required effective monitoring of trends and family planning strategies that took account of the population impact. A comparatively new phenomenon in an increasing number of countries of the region was the growing quantum of female migration, including migration of single women. A better understanding of the demographic, economic and social implications of such migration was essential. The management of metropolitan cities was another issue that deserved high priority. In several countries, the growth rate of large cities had slackened. Small cities were suffering from stagnation and obsolescence while medium-size cities were expanding rapidly. Spatial implications and environmental consequences of major sectoral policies should be fully assessed as part of the national development planning process to achieve balanced urbanization, keeping in mind the objective of reducing rural-urban disparities, regional disparities within countries and the need to protect the environment. To cope with rapid urbanization, Governments should create a favourable climate for private sector investment in smaller towns and cities and provide the required support mechanisms, such as physical and social infrastructure and advantageous fiscal and monetary policies.

The Bali Conference was also concerned that while the proportion of older persons remained low in many ESCAP countries, the absolute number of older persons was swelling. The trends and patterns in population movements had further added to the ageing of rural areas, as those who migrated to urban areas tended to be young and able, leaving behind the elderly to attend to farming and other agricultural pursuits, thus adversely affecting agricultural production. Hence, migration had to be closely monitored and redirected by creating job opportunities and other incentives for the young to remain in rural areas. The Conference stressed the need to create awareness of ageing issues and provide the necessary incentives for families to continue caring for their elderly. Emphasis was laid on strengthening community support through the formation of voluntary and mutual aid organizations; encouraging communities to provide the necessary services for elderly care and integrating older persons into all aspects of development; establishing appropriate home industries that enabled the elderly to work at their own pace; and initiating training programmes to improve the productivity of the elderly and their continued participation in the advancement of new technologies and industries.

The population of countries and areas comprising the ESCAP region reached 3.7 billion in the year 2000, i.e., double the population 40 years earlier, and accounting for approximately 62 per cent of the world's population. Fertility levels were diminishing in almost all countries of the region because of family planning services provided under government programmes, among other factors. The Fifth APPC noted that many developing countries in the region were characterized by overpopulation, poverty, malnutrition, poor health and inadequate and unsustainable health-care financing. While economic growth was essential for development and poverty reduction, lowering fertility and population growth rates was equally important in that regard. There was increasing evidence to indicate that the alterations in age structure taking place in most countries could contribute significantly to economic growth if appropriate policies were put in place such as pro-poor economic and social policies that promoted choice; enhanced the development of, access to and utilization of resources; improved gender equity and equality; and increased access to reproductive health, including family planning.

Adolescent reproductive health information and service programmes were still in the early stages of development, were too narrowly focused and were not adequately available to adolescents in general and unmarried adolescents in particular, with young people not often involved in programme planning and development. The Conference strongly supported the right of young people to adolescent reproductive health, especially as a means for preventing unwanted pregnancies, abortion and the spread of HIV/AIDS. The delegations observed that where social, cultural or religious barriers existed to prevent young people from obtaining information on sexual matters at home, sex education and training in life skills should be provided for young people in and outside the school systems, especially in view of their exposure to conflicting forms of information on sexual matters through the media, pornographic sites on the Internet and the popularity of its unmoderated electronic "chat rooms". Behavioural change communication, advocacy and education programmes should be implemented to raise awareness and enhance communication with parents, families, teachers, religious and community leaders, service providers and other adults, peer groups and mass media on improved reproductive health for adolescents.

Many Asian and Pacific countries assessed the existing policy environment and resource base for mainstreaming gender concerns, established national machineries and focal points and developed national plans of action for improving the status of women. While substantial progress had been demonstrated through improved education, health status and labour force participation of females, the gains were unequal among the countries of the region. Although the gender gap had narrowed somewhat in terms of gross enrolment at the primary level, the female disadvantage persisted at the higher educational levels in almost all countries and areas of the region. The share of female wage employment in the non-agricultural sector was low and the proportion of seats held by women in parliaments remained under 10 per cent, on average. Emerging issues in the region included the marginalization of female employment, the rise in poor female-headed households, increase in girl-child labour and trafficking of women and children. Governments in cooperation with civil society organizations and the international community were urged to reduce the marginalization of women in employment through policies and programmes that addressed gender-based discrimination and also reduced the negative impact of globalization on women's employment while recognizing its positive impact in empowering women and augmenting opportunities in decision-making. Exploitation of children could be eliminated through vigorous policy actions and their effective implementation. Awareness of gender-based violence should be increased, relevant laws simplified and law enforcement officials trained to ensure the effective enforcement of adequate and appropriate legislative and programmatic responses to violence against women and exploitation, including trafficking. Policies should be formulated to promote greater male involvement and participation in improving gender equality, equity and empowerment of women.

Role of the United Nations, ECAFE and ESCAP

At its 1964 session, the Commission unanimously adopted resolution 54 (XX) of 17 March 1964, in which it requested the secretariat to expand its activities in particular fields of work relating to the population problems of the region. Subsequently, the Economic and Social Council adopted resolution 1048 (XXXVII) in August 1964, commending ECAFE for organizing the First APC and drawing the attention of the General Assembly to the Commission's resolution. ECAFE continued to be the focal point among countries and areas in the region in the population dialogue and in population information dissemination. The Commission members welcomed the secretariat's work in family planning and in the relationship between population and agricultural change.

The secretariat played a central role in initiating debate on population and development issues in the region, providing the forum for the region's developing countries to address them and assisting those countries through its regional programmes, advisory services, training and information dissemination activities. The Bali Conference called upon ESCAP to continue to play a pivotal role in assisting members and associate members in implementing their population and development policies and programmes. It recommended that ESCAP fully incorporate the population dimension into the focus of three thematic committees: regional economic cooperation, environment and sustainable development and poverty alleviation.

The capacity of the United Nations system to provide assistance to countries was increased as a result of the establishment of the United Nations Fund for Population Activities (UNFPA) in 1967. Its resources through voluntary contributions from countries grew from US$ 7 million in 1970 to nearly US$ 40 million in 1972. Those funds were available for projects related to all aspects of population, including family planning programmes in developing countries. The extension of the UNFPA system of country coordinators, together with the United Nations Development Programme's newly instituted system of country programming, helped to prevent duplication of effort and of measures that were not mutually supporting. UNFPA had taken steps to increase its administrative capacity to respond more effectively to requests for assistance from Commission members for the design and implementation of their population policies in accordance with national priorities, working closely with government officials to ensure effective coordination and harmonization of population activities and to develop fully national capacity for self-reliance. UNFPA assisted ESCAP in playing an enhanced role in helping developing countries in the region to shape their future population policies and programmes.

Since 1990, the ESCAP region has been the second-largest recipient of population assistance after sub-Saharan Africa. According to UNFPA, final expenditures for population assistance in the region increased from US$ 211.5 million in 1990 to US$ 389.3 million in the year 2000. The bilateral and multilateral channels each accounted for over 30 per cent of funds expended in the region. A total of 39 countries and territories in the region benefited from international population assistance in 2000 with Bangladesh, India and the Philippines as the top three recipient countries. A total of US$ 19.5 million was spent on regional programmes.

Appropriate steps have been taken to reorient the Asian and Pacific regional programme on population and sustainable development with a view to assisting developing countries in the region, paying special attention to least developed countries, in response to the challenges that they face and the need to strengthen national capacity. In that regard, ESCAP staff members have provided technical assistance to a large number of members and associate members of the Commission on a wide range of population and reproductive health issues during the years since the adoption of the resolution 54/4 on 22 April 1998. Such assistance has included policy and programme development, capacity-building, the collection and analysis of data from censuses and surveys, detailed analysis of and research on priority issues, as well as programme monitoring and evaluation of population and reproductive health programmes. Staff members of ESCAP have acted as resource persons for intercountry workshops on population and reproductive health issues organized by the secretariat, the Statistical Institute for Asia and the Pacific, the UNFPA Country Technical Services Team for East and South-East Asia, Chulalongkorn University in Thailand and the Asian Forum of Parliamentarians on Population and Development. A considerable number of seminars, expert group meetings and training workshops have been organized for capacity development in the region on various aspects of population and development and for maximizing the benefits of modern information technologies for processing and disseminating data and information.

Reflections

From the First APC in 1963 to the Fifth APPC in 2002, the Conferences have dealt with population concerns at the regional and global levels. The purposes of the Conferences, the themes, the agenda items taken up during the successive meetings and the resolutions and plans of action adopted by delegations at each Conference all reflected the predominant population and development issues at the time.

What is striking is the strong will and collaboration shown by the Commission's members and associate members in tackling what they perceived to be critical demographic problems and in arriving at pertinent solutions. The technical and financial support of the United Nations, its specialized agencies and UNFPA, enabled member States to embark on family planning and reproductive health programmes to achieve their population and development goals.

The Fifth APPC revealed the dramatic reversal in thinking of the Government of the United States of America since the 1994 ICPD. While the United States actively supported the paradigm shift to reproductive health in Cairo, the change of administration in the year 2000 has led to its vigorous campaign against reaffirming the ICPD Programme of Action in toto, objecting to such terms as reproductive health, reproductive health services and adolescent reproductive health in the belief that these terms promote abortion and underage sex. Thus, the United States delegation attempted to substantially revise or to block the adoption of the draft Plan of Action during the Fifth APPC. This caused the other delegations to take a unified stand to reaffirm the ICPD Programme of Action. If the United States stand remains unaltered in the coming decade, holding a 10-year review and appraisal of ICPD (ICPD+10) or a Sixth APPC would likely be an exercise in futility.

It is imperative that the population community sustain its efforts to keep the population perspective in the forefront of issues such as globalization, environment and sustainable development even if the Plan of Action in these areas ignores population, as was patently obvious at the 2002 World Summit on Sustainable Development held at Johannesburg, South Africa. By reiterating its affirmation of the relevant international conventions, by vigorously lobbying at international forums and by supporting regional collaboration in population and development programmes, the population community underscores the importance of maintaining the population perspective in the discussion of issues germane to genuine development.

Endnote

This paper was based on the reports of each of the five Asian (and Pacific) Population Conferences held since 1963 and the papers prepared by the secretariat and UNFPA for the Fifth APPC.

The Fifth Asian and Pacific Population Conference: Towards a Repositioning of Population in the Global Development Agenda?

*There is an urgent need to reposition population
in the global development agenda. In doing so, the first point
to make is that people's welfare is the ultimate objective
of all development planning*

By Gavin Jones*

Antecedents to the Bangkok Conference

The Fifth Asian and Pacific Population Conference, held at Bangkok in December 2002, followed a little more than 10 years after the Fourth Asian and

* Professor, Research School of Social Sciences, Australian National University, Canberra, Australia, e-mail: Gavin.Jones@anu.edu.au

Pacific Population Conference, held at Bali. The Bali Conference was one of the regional conferences leading up to the path-breaking International Conference on Population and Development, held at Cairo in 1994, and was important in the context of providing input into the Cairo Conference, but also in its own right as reflecting the consensus among the Member States making up over 60 per cent of the world's population.

It is well known that the Cairo Conference led to some dramatic shifts in direction in the rhetoric of population and development, as well as in the priorities for and conduct of national population programmes. These shifts in direction had not been apparent at the Bali Conference, which had indeed spelled out a set of population targets in line with sustainable development goals, an approach that came under attack from various sources at Cairo (McIntosh and Finkle 1995: 227). The Cairo document, in paragraphs 3.14, 3.25, 3.26, 3.28, 6.3 and 6.4, gives muted support to the need to reduce population growth rates. But the main thrust of the document lies elsewhere. "Population policy becomes a welfarist activity, seeking especially to benefit women. Effects on birth rates are not so much seen as secondary, but as an inevitable – and desired – consequence of women's empowerment" (McNicoll 1995: 334).

The emphasis on reproductive health and reproductive rights was a major accomplishment of the Cairo Conference, though the stress on women's empowerment was arguably taken too far in some areas: for example, by stressing gender inequities in access to education while ignoring inequities in access by socio-economic status (Knodel and Jones 1996) and viewing the gender difference in child mortality as "much more crucial than the high level of child mortality, male and female, in poor societies across the world" (Basu 1997: 226). Be that as it may, the countries and areas of the ESCAP region, individually and as a group, made concerted efforts to orient their policies and programmes to the new emphases of Cairo. This was evident, for example, in the stress placed on adolescent reproductive health in the report of the high-level meeting held at Bangkok in 1998 to review the implementation of the Cairo Programme of Action and the earlier Bali Declaration on Population and Sustainable Development (ESCAP 1998). Adolescent reproductive health had been ignored in the Bali document.

In the decade that passed between the Fourth and the Fifth Asian and Pacific Population Conferences, the world (and specifically the Asian and Pacific region) had moved on, in terms of both its economic and demographic situations. First of all, the demographic transition in the region had progressed considerably. This can be observed by comparing the total fertility rate and expectation of life at birth in the region at the time of the two Conferences. In 1992, these were about 3.1 and 63 years, respectively. In 2002, they had fallen to about 2.6 and risen to about 67 years, respectively. Not only this, but by 2002 there were few countries where fertility had not started to decline. In 1992, real doubts could still be raised about whether any decline had taken place in Cambodia, Nepal or Pakistan. By 2002 they could not.

At the other end of the spectrum, by 2002, some countries where fertility in 1992 was already below replacement level had sunk to even lower levels, and the implications of this low fertility were causing considerable concern. In general, then, demographically the Asian and Pacific region had become even more diverse than it had been in 1992, but with a clear shift towards lower fertility and mortality levels. Although demographic momentum was clearly going to swell population numbers very considerably, the overriding need to lower fertility rates, which had been recognized in the Asian and Pacific Population Conferences of the 1970s and 1980s, and indeed to a lesser though still substantial extent in 1992, was no longer such a priority concern in 2002.

In terms of economic development, the decade had seen impressive growth in the Asian and Pacific region, albeit with considerable variation. Population and poverty was appropriately chosen as the theme of the Bangkok Conference, but this did not mean that the incidence of poverty was getting worse. Indeed, a recent Asian Development Bank study of 18 Asian countries, using national poverty lines and survey estimates of consumption, found that the poverty incidence in these countries had fallen from 65 per cent in 1960 to 17 per cent in 2000. The biggest decline came during the last two decades.[1] Major countries in the region – China, Indonesia, Thailand and Viet Nam– have seen major reductions in the incidence of poverty (Jones 2002: 6-9). Though there can be (and are) debates about the exact trends, there can be no contesting the reality of a substantial decline in the incidence of poverty in all these countries. Even the Asian economic crisis, which hit countries including Indonesia, the Republic of Korea and Thailand hard from 1997, was not able to put a major dint in the general reduction in poverty throughout the region. Africa was the continent where poverty increases were matters of grave concern; the Asian and Pacific region was certainly not Africa.

The thrust of the Bangkok Conference

The debate at the Bangkok Conference reflected the continuing vital interest of the countries and areas of the Asian and Pacific region in the interrelationships between population trends and development. Many of these countries had espoused the Programme of Action of the Cairo Conference with a degree of diffidence, recognizing the winds of change that were seemingly unstoppable at that Conference, yet concerned that their continuing strong national emphases on reducing fertility rates through family planning and other measures would be undermined by the new emphasis on reproductive health and reproductive rights. Since that time, debates have continued throughout the region about the degree of compatibility of reproductive health approaches with the aim of lowering fertility, with some protagonists arguing that by diluting family planning resources, the impacts on fertility will weaken, and others making the point that a well-executed reproductive health approach will lower dropout and failure rates and appeal to those younger people whose delayed sexual initiation and longer and effective practice of contraception are crucial to a sustained decline in fertility. However, as noted earlier, demographic trends have reduced the salience of efforts to reduce fertility in many of the Asian and Pacific countries, and for this reason alone, leaving aside changes in the ideology of family planning and reproductive health, reducing fertility is no longer as prominent a concern of the region as it was at the time of the Bali Conference.

There are many issues surrounding reproductive health and reproductive rights, apart from their relation to fertility reduction strategies. At the Cairo Conference, certain of the Asian and Pacific countries shared the concern of some other countries that the sections on reproductive health and reproductive rights in the Cairo Programme of Action might have the effect of promoting abortion or adolescent sexual activity. However, many of them were more concerned that the protracted debate over these issues at Cairo served to constrict discussion of the kinds of broader population and development issues that had received considerable attention at the Bali Conference. On this score, history repeated itself in Bangkok. An inordinate proportion of the time of the drafting committee was taken up with the concerns of the United States of America delegation about language contained in the Cairo Programme of Action, which according to that delegation, tended to promote abortion and adolescent sexual activity. In the event, the Asian and Pacific countries stood firm in supporting the language of the Cairo Programme of Action (the cohesion of such a diverse group of countries in doing so being one of the most striking features of the Conference), but at the cost of minimizing the time and intellectual effort that could be devoted to other important aspects of the Plan of Action.

It is clear that as time has moved on, the Cairo consensus has become entrenched in Asian and Pacific countries' approaches to population issues, and nowhere is this seen better than in these countries' determination to adhere to the language contained in the Cairo Programme of Action in the Plan of Action finally agreed to at Bangkok. Country delegation after country delegation, in statements from the floor, indicated their conviction that the Cairo consensus did not in any way promote abortion or adolescent sexual activity.

Though the debates in Bangkok were focused heavily on this issue, if we examine the Plan of Action on Population and Poverty that was adopted by consensus at the conclusion of the Conference, it does have a great deal to say about population and development. In this sense, it will serve as a benchmark for policy emphases for some time.

What are the main emphases of the Plan of Action? First of all, in terms of overall directions, the preamble emphasizes the centrality of poverty eradication concerns and recognizes that sustainable development requires an appropriate balance between economic growth, poverty, resources and environment. The preamble recognizes the importance of human capital and in that context refers to the special need to address women's disadvantage and marginalization. Human rights are recognized as central to development and population policies are seen as an integral component of development policies and planning. The preamble then indicates that these concerns are in line with previous consensus by the international community by affirming a commitment to the principles and recommendations adopted in Bali, Cairo, Beijing (Fourth World Conference on Women), five-year review reports on Bali and Cairo, and finally the Millennium Declaration.

As for the strategic recommendations of the Plan of Action, these are set out under 12 headings:

> Population, sustainable development and poverty
> International migration
> Internal migration and urbanization
> Population ageing
> Gender equality, equity and empowerment of women
> Reproductive rights and reproductive health
> Adolescent reproductive health
> HIV/AIDS
> Behavioural change communication and information and
>   communication technology
> Data, research and training
> Partnerships
> Resources

In the end, the reader of the document will find it to be carefully worded, reflecting current consensus about principles and broad directions for action in these important areas, and not distorted by the highly skewed amounts of time spent in debating and discussing certain sections. In this respect, it reflects the considerable work that had gone into drafting the document, large sections of which were able to be adopted by consensus without need for lengthy discussion.

The difficulty of reaching a consensus at Bangkok actually reflected, not divisions within the ESCAP members, but rather their determination to maintain the commitment to the principles and recommendations of earlier Conferences, most notably the Cairo Conference, when that was challenged by one delegation. The publicity given to this issue was described in a statement by the Asian Forum of Parliamentarians on Population and Development as creating "such hype that population has received new energy" (<http://www.afppd.org/informat.htm>). Is this just hyperbole, or will a new impetus be given to population concerns as a result of the Bangkok Conference? It is really too early to judge, and a balanced assessment will need to be based on the actions of individual countries, groupings of countries and donor agencies over the coming years. Nevertheless, it is appropriate at least to look for "straws in the wind" at this stage.

What is the general outlook for the field of population now?

The 10-year review and appraisal of ICPD, also known as ICPD +10, is due to be held in 2004. If it is indeed held, the context will be different from that of the Cairo Conference. One of the key differences is that population growth rates are slowing quite generally throughout the world. Not only this, but many countries are now very concerned about excessively low fertility, which will lead in time to a significant downward spiral in population size unless fertility rates can be raised.

The steam has really gone out of the population issue as conventionally understood. Though world population is still expected to grow from the current 6.2 billion to somewhere between 7.3 and 10.4 billion by 2050, the growth will be at ever-decreasing rates. There is now said to be a 60 per cent probability that the world's population will not exceed 10 billion people before 2100 (Lutz, Sanderson and Scherbov 2001: 543), a far cry from earlier projections which suggested the likelihood of considerably larger populations (see also Bongaarts and Bulatao, eds. 2000). Though the need to lower birth rates is still of critical importance in some countries, particularly in Africa and South Asia, nobody seems to doubt any more that these declines will take place.

Popular attention, as guided by the emphases in the news media, has turned to issues that are considered more pressing, in particular, issues of environmental sustainability and poverty. Donor agencies, foundations and universities have likewise moved on to issues that they see as more on the "cutting edge", matters including environment and poverty, and post-11 September terrorism. Some of them see illegal migration and refugee movements, both of them "population issues",- as issues of considerable moment.

The general understanding that population issues are a thing of the past is unfortunate for two reasons. First, population and development issues are just as important for countries with low fertility as they are for countries with high fertility. Dealing with changing age structures and declining populations presents formidable intellectual and planning challenges. Secondly, there are important population dimensions of the issues that are currently given greatest prominence (see, for example, Geist and Lambin 2002 on population and the environment), but these dimensions are insufficiently recognized by the agencies dealing with them (for example, population was effectively ignored at the World Summit on Sustainable Development, held at Johannesburg in 2002).

In other words, academics, planners, international agencies and NGOs concerned with population and development issues have not "sold" the population field very effectively, and we are now suffering the consequences. Thirty or 40 years ago, when population growth appeared almost out of control, it was easy to see population as an area of crucial importance. But at that time, most university population programmes, international agencies and foundations dealing with population issues were content to ride the wave of popular concern, without devoting enough attention to educating the public to the crucial demographic dimensions of planning issues, whether in circumstances of rapid population growth or of slower or even negative population growth. Perhaps the greatest indictment of population researchers and planners is that we have been too ready to espouse one-dimensional notions of the adverse impacts of rapid population growth on development, without acknowledging that population trends – and the way in which they impact on society and development – are influenced by the complex sociocultural and political settings in which they occur. It is somewhat ironic that we are now claiming that population itself is being left out of the equation by those from other disciplines when assessing the causes of poverty or environmental degradation.

Trends in institutional and financial support

What does the flow of international development assistance indicate about the importance of the field of population nowadays? Is population being marginalized in the broad context of development assistance?

First, it needs to be noted that the agreed international goals for official development assistance (ODA), i.e., a proportion of 0.7 per cent of the GNP of the wealthy countries, have never been reached, or indeed ever approached. Although reiterated in the Millennium Declaration adopted by the Member States of the United Nations at the Millennium Summit in September 2000, the lack of demonstrated will to reach this goal in practice, at a time of rising expenditures on armaments and security, is one of the most depressing facts of our time. "Compassion fatigue" appears to have become a permanent state of enervation in the wealthier countries. The specification, in the Monterrey Consensus adopted at the International Conference on Financing for Development in 2002, of the need for the adoption of sound policies and good governance in developing countries to ensure the effective use of ODA implicitly acknowledges one of the reasons for such "compassion fatigue". Unfortunately, it does not necessarily follow that improvements in this direction by the developing countries will loosen the purse strings in developed countries.

As for population activities specifically, many attempts were made, even before Cairo, to come up with estimates of the costs of population programmes. Estimates of global resources needed in the year 2000 ranged widely, between US$ 600 million (for just contraceptive commodities) to US$ 11.5 billion (see Zeitlin, Govindaraj and Chen 1994). This highlights one of the problems in tracking how much has really been devoted to meeting the goals of the Cairo Conference: the boundaries of population spending are very hard to define, once broader reproductive health becomes the key objective, and even more so if recognition is given to the demographic impacts of spending on broader areas such as education.

The ICPD Programme of Action specified the financial resources, both domestic and donor funded, believed necessary to implement a wide-ranging population and reproductive health package. For the year 2000, the estimate was US$ 17 billion (US$ 11 billion in the ESCAP region), rising to US$ 18.5 billion by 2005. Approximately two thirds were expected to come from domestic sources and one third from the international donor community (UNFPA 2002). Subsequent UNFPA monitoring of international population assistance and domestic spending for population activities shows that financial constraints remain one of the chief obstacles to the realization of the ICPD objectives. According to UNFPA estimates, the total sum generated in 1999-2000 was about US$ 11 billion, with international population assistance funds (which reached only about 46 per cent of the target) falling further short of the target than domestically generated funds (UNFPA 2002). Given the ESCAP region's large share of total required funds, it is clear that the relative shortfall within the ESCAP region must be of the same general order of magnitude as the overall shortfall.

Such broad-grained estimates of funding shortfalls are really of questionable relevance when the complex determinants of population trends are recognized. What other points can be made about the relative importance accorded population issues, especially in the Asian and Pacific region, in the post-Bangkok Conference world?

It would be easy to seize on the downgrading of population activities in ESCAP (already in train before the Bangkok Conference), as well as a shrinking of resources provided by UNFPA, as signs that population issues are no longer as high up on the priority list of development issues as they once were. However, the Asian Development Bank and the World Bank seem to be continuing a substantial level of support for population projects. Although the United States Government cut off support for UNFPA in 2002, this does not mean that it is reducing its support for population programmes, but just redirecting it to other ways of financing those population activities that meet its ideological conditions.

The situation regarding population data is a mixed bag. On the plus side, demographic and health surveys have provided many Asian countries with a sound basis for assessing trends in and determinants of fertility and mortality, for many of them at more than one date, but few Asian and Pacific countries can track annual changes in fertility and mortality from vital registration data. And the problems faced by many countries of the region with their 2000 round of population censuses seem to reflect not only country-specific issues such as the impact of governmental decentralization in Indonesia and the Philippines, but also a squeezing of funds which, even in these times of financial stress, reflects the lowly place in the financial priorities spectrum accorded population data. Population data received more attention when it seemed crucial to know just how rapid population growth rates were, and whether efforts to bring them down were succeeding.

What might be done to follow up on the Plan of Action adopted in Bangkok?

There is an urgent need to reposition population in the global development agenda. In doing so, the first point to make is that people's welfare is the ultimate objective of all development planning. Therefore, we need to know who those people are in the aggregate – what are their characteristics, and the trends in the composition of this population. The second point is that there are demographic components of all aspects of development planning – in all settings, not just those where rapid population growth is seen as a problem. The difficulty of showing precisely how population dynamics are implicated in the key issues of current concern, such as poverty and the environment, should be seen as a challenge to the demographic community rather than a reason to be silent. It behoves the population community in the region to use its influence in a range of settings – government deliberations, planning meetings, seminars and through the media – to drive home the point that population matters.

This implies the need for a good understanding of demographic trends, which in turn implies the need for good data and good research. Increased spending on demographic data collection is vital, as is adequate support for demographic programmes in universities, including programmes emphasizing interactions between demographic and socio-economic trends. Adequate data and research capacity should be seen as the building blocks for an effective understanding of population issues.

Finally, the Cairo emphasis, reiterated at Bangkok, requires continuing attention to reproductive health issues. There are still a tragically large number of people having children they do not want, and also some who are not able to have children they would like to have. There are unconscionably high maternal mortality rates in many Asian and Pacific countries, and millions whose lives are blighted by non-life threatening sexually transmitted diseases and reproductive tract infections. In this context, unmet need and a balanced understanding of its causes should remain a key pillar of family planning approaches (Sinding and others 1994; Casterline and Sinding 2000). Pilot projects are needed to test reproductive health approaches that work, but perhaps even more necessary at this stage is analysis of ways to scale up successful pilot or experimental projects to the larger programmatic settings in which reproductive health services will be provided, beset by the usual problems of large-scale bureaucracies (Simmons, Brown and Diaz 2002). To bring effective reproductive health facilities to poorer countries requires money, planning and changed attitudes on the part of both those who determine government budgets and many health providers. Serious and imaginative attention to these issues will not only ensure lower population growth rates in countries where these remain troublingly high, but will also have major benefits for quality of life.

Endnote

1.   While not denying the reality of these declines, it needs to be noted that the inclusion of an estimate of those living in "near poverty" would raise the poverty group to considerably higher numbers, as many national poverty lines measure mere "survival-level" existence.

References

Basu, Alaka (1997). "The new international population movement: a framework for a constructive critique", *Health Transition Review*, vol. 7, Supplement 4.

Bongaarts, J. and R. Bulatao, eds. (2000). *Beyond Six Billion: Forecasting the World's Population* (Washington, The National Academies Press).

Casterline, John B. and Steven W. Sinding (2000). "Unmet need for family planning in developing countries and implications for population policy", *Population and Development Review*, vol. 26, No. 4, pp. 691-723.

ESCAP (1998). *Asia-Pacific Population Policies and Programmes: Future Directions -- Report, Key Future Actions and Background Papers of a High-level Meeting*, Asian Population Studies Series No. 153, (United Nations publication, Sales No.E.99.II.F.4).

Geist, Helmut J. and Eric F. Lambin. (2002). "Proximate causes and underlying driving forces of tropical deforestation", *BioScience*, vol. 52, No. 2, pp. 143-150.

Jones, Gavin W. (2002). "Population and poverty in Asia and the Pacific", paper presented at the Fifth Asian and Pacific Population Conference, Senior Officials Segment, Bangkok, 11-14 December.

Knodel, John and Gavin W. Jones (1996). "Post-Cairo population policy: does promoting girls' schooling miss the mark?", *Population and Development Review*, vol. 22, No.4 , pp. 683-702.

Lutz, Wolfgang, Warren Sanderson and Sergei Scherbov (2001). "The end of world population growth", *Nature*, vol. 412, pp. 543-545.

McIntosh, C. Alison and Jason L. Finkle (1995). "The Cairo Conference on Population and Development: a new paradigm?", *Population and Development Review*, vol. 21, No. 2, pp. 223-260.

McNicoll, Geoffrey (1995). "On population growth and revisionism: further questions", *Population and Development Review*, vol. 21, No. 2, pp. 307-340.

Simmons, Ruth, Joseph Brown and Margarita Diaz (2002). "Facilitating large-scale transitions to quality of care: an idea whose time has come", *Studies in Family Planning*, vol. 33, No. 1, pp. 61-75.

Sinding, Stephen W., John A. Ross and Allan G. Rosenfield (1994). "Seeking common ground: unmet need and demographic goals", *International Family Planning Perspectives,* vol. 20, No. 1, pp. 23-29.

UNFPA (2002). "Resource mobilization in the ESCAP region", paper presented at the Fifth Asian and Pacific Population Conference, Senior Officials Segment, Bangkok, 11-14 December.

Zeitlin, Jennifer, Ramesh Govindaraj and Lincoln C. Chen (1994). "Financing reproductive and sexual health services", in Gita Sen, Adrienne Germain and Lincoln C. Chen, eds., *Population Policies Reconsidered: Health, Empowerment, and Rights* (Harvard, Harvard University Press).

Knowledge of Sexual Health Issues among Unmarried Young People in Nepal

*In the context of a global decline in age of sexual maturation
and rising age of marriage, the window of opportunity for young people
to engage in premarital sexual relations is opening*

By Nicole Stone, Roger Ingham and Padam Simkhada*

Early and universal marriage has traditionally been the norm in Nepalese culture, although the practise of delayed marriage appears to be on the increase. In 1961, nearly 75 per cent of young women aged 15 to19 years were married; this

* Nicole Stone, Research Fellow, Centre for Sexual Health Research, Department of Social Statistics, University of Southampton, Highfield, Southampton, SO17 1BJ, United Kingdom of Great Britain and Northern Ireland, e-mail: ncs@socsci.soton.ac.uk; Roger Ingham, Reader in Health and Community Psychology, Director, Centre for Sexual Health Research, Department of Psychology, University of Southampton, Highfield, Southampton, SO17 1BJ, United Kingdom, e-mail: ri@soton.ac.uk; Padam Simkhada, Research Fellow, Department of Public Health, University of Aberdeen, Foresterhill, Aberdeen AB25 2ZD Scotland, United Kingdom, e-mail: p.p.simkhada@abdn.ac.uk

figure declined to just under 50 per cent by 1991 and to a low of 40 per cent in 2001 (Mehta 1998; Khanal 1999; NDHS 1996 and 2001). This, along with the advent of reducing age at first menarche due to improved nutritional status, has led to an increase in the window of opportunity for premarital sexual activity to occur.

Owing to social and cultural taboos and inhibitions, sexual health research in Nepal remains restricted to a small number of studies; for young people, especially those who are unmarried, this is particularly pertinent. Further, much of the hitherto limited research with young people remains unpublished.

Findings from studies which have investigated premarital sexual behaviour among high school and college students have found rates of activity to vary from 11 per cent among students in Pokhara to 14 per cent among Kathmandu students [1] and 16 per cent among students[1] in Palpa District (Limbu 2001; Prasai 1999). Among young unmarried men and women aged 14 to 19 years working in factories in the Kathmandu Valley, 20 per cent and 12 per cent of the men and women respectively reported having experienced sex (Puri 2002). Further, studies of single men in the border towns of Nepal found activity rates of 10 per cent among a sample aged 15 to 19 years and about 50 per cent among a slightly older sample aged 18 to 24 years (Mehta 1998; Tamang and others 2001).

Although the use of modern contraceptives in Nepal has risen steadily over the last two decades, levels still remain low (NDHS 2001; Pradhan and others 1997). For example, among currently married women, ever use and current use of a modern method stand at 50 and 35 per cent respectively. The use of condoms also remains particularly low at only 3 per cent for current usage and 12 per cent for ever use, rising to a high of only 16 per cent among women aged 20 to 24 years (NDHS 2001). Given the perceived problems associated with the discussion of personal sexual behaviour outside of marriage, there is a dearth of information with regard to safer sexual practices during premarital and extramarital sex. A study of condom use during sex with non-regular partners by married and unmarried young men (18 to 24 years), however, found that just over half had used a condom during the last intercourse (Tamang and others 2001). Furthermore, in the light of rising rates of sexually transmitted infections (STIs) among certain target groups and increasing rates of unplanned pregnancies, leading to maternal morbidity and mortality from unsafe abortions, it would appear that safer-sex practices during premarital and extramarital relations are infrequently being adhered to (Dahal 1999; Furber and others 2002; Mehta 1998; UNFPA 1996).

Data collected during the demographic and health surveys as well as from small-scale surveys indicate that awareness of condoms, HIV/AIDS and other STIs appears to be rising among the general population, mainly owing to extensive media campaigns (NDHS 1996 and 2001; Mehta 1998; Pradhan and others 1997). In 2000, the Nepal Adolescent and Young Adults Survey (NAYA) questioned both married and unmarried young people (aged 14 to 22 years) regarding their awareness of contraception and HIV/AIDS. Their results showed that 93 per cent of young people had heard of HIV/AIDS and 95 per cent were aware of condoms (Neupane and Nichols 2002; Aryal and Nichols 2002).

For many young people in Nepal, however, especially those who are unmarried, social and cultural norms impose barriers to the transfer of sexual health information. Consequently, countless remain ignorant of even the basic knowledge required for safer sexual behaviour. For example, when the comprehensiveness of knowledge was tested during the NAYA survey, among those young people who had ever heard of HIV/AIDS, only 36 per cent were able to cite all three of the following measures to reduce or avoid the possibility of exposure: avoiding sex with a prostitute, using a condom during sex and having one steady partner (Neupane and Nichols 2002). Further, among young people who were aware of condoms, 1 in 10 did not know they could be used to protect against pregnancy, including 1 in 6 married young women.

Evidence from other country settings shows that sex education delivered in school can make a positive contribution to children and young people's knowledge and personal and social development, helping to prevent negative health outcomes such as unintended pregnancies and STIs. It contributes to preparing pupils for the opportunities, responsibilities and experiences of adult life and, when linked to confidential sexual health services, is shown to delay the onset of sexual activity. To achieve sustainable change, however, it is necessary to focus on young people before they become sexually active, before myths become deep-rooted and unsafe patterns of sexual behaviour are established (Kirby 2001; Grunseit and others 1997).

Nepal's education policies over the last 30 years, including the provision of free education up to secondary level, scholarship programmes for girls and the launching of the Education for All campaign, have greatly increased school attendance and raised the educational status of both males and females. In 1998, Nepal had 58,000 trained and 72,000 untrained teachers teaching more than 4.8 million students in 34,000 primary and secondary schools (Nepal 1998). Schools therefore have the potential to act as a key resource in the struggle to achieve optimal sexual health among Nepal's young people.

The present secondary school education curriculum includes health, population and environmental education as a compulsory subject in classes 9 and 10; topics covered include reproductive health, family life education and safe motherhood. Additionally there are two optional courses on health education and population education. Anecdotal evidence suggests, however, that classes, where they are taught, tend to be biomedical in focus, teaching methods tend to be didactic and time allocation is limited. To date, insufficient research has focused on investigating the quality of sexuality education within the school context in Nepal, although some pilot work has been undertaken (Prasai 1999).

In the light of the need to provide high-quality sex education in schools, the Department for International Development (DFID)-funded Safe Paassages to Adulthood programme (based at the University of Southampton, United Kingdom) funded the local non-governmental organization, The Society for Local Integrated Development Nepal (SOLID Nepal) to investigate the challenges facing Nepal in its development of a more comprehensive sex and sexuality education curriculum in secondary schools. Using a combination of qualitative and quantitative research techniques, information was gained on young people's, teachers' and parents' knowledge, experiences and attitudes towards school-based sex education, perceived barriers to improving the curriculum and opportunities for change. This paper presents some of the findings from the questionnaire survey conducted among high school students, in particular, the sections focusing on sources of information and current knowledge of sexual health matters.

Methodology

The research consisted of a quantitative self-completion questionnaire distributed among young people attending school in classes 8, 9 and 10.[2] Section 1 covered basic demographic questions including age, sex, family composition, parental education and employment status, ethnicity, religion and, as measured by provision of household amenities and assets, socio-economic status. Section 2 asked respondents about their current sources of information about sexual and reproductive health and assessed knowledge. Section 3 asked pupils' views and attitudes concerning a series of health and sexuality issues, and section 4 focused on the sex and sexuality education the respondents had received at school, including issues discussed, teaching methods used, quality of teaching, improvements that could be made and other relevant issues. This paper explores factors that influence young people's sexual health knowledge.

Three districts, out of a total of 75 in Nepal, were purposively selected for distribution of the questionnaire; Dhading, Morang and Lalitpur. The sites were selected to represent regions of differential development, urban, semi-urban and rural settings and cultural and ethnic diversity.

Dhading district is located in the Central Development Region of Nepal and borders China. The district consists of remote communities with limited access to electricity and telephones. Road access is poor with the only motorable road linking the district headquarters with Kathmandu being five hours' drive away. Morang district is located in the Terai in the Eastern Development Region bordering India. Electricity and telephones are available here, although not comprehensively. Finally, Lalitpur is the second biggest city of Nepal and located within the Kathmandu Valley. It is located in the Central Development Region and is one of the most urbanized cities. Communication facilities are extensive and include national and international television, fax, telex and the Internet. Residents in Lalitpur are widely exposed to the tourist trade and the district has a diverse cultural mix.

Owing to political, access and communication barriers it was not possible to undertake a fully random sample of schools in the selected areas. Therefore, purposive sampling techniques were employed. Suitable high school educational establishments in the three sites were contacted by the research team and invited to participate in the research. From those who agreed, three schools in Lalitpur, two in Morang and one in Dhading were chosen and issued with questionnaires to be distributed among pupils in the target classes. The final selection of schools was proportionate to the number of secondary schools in each district and all, except one in Lalitpur, were government-run.[3]

The questionnaires were based on an appropriately adapted version of a questionnaire previously used in another country context to examine quality of sex education. Following pre-testing, 1,200 questionnaires were distributed in the six educational establishments. After obtaining written consent and giving oral instructions on how to complete the questionnaire, forms were filled in under the supervision of a researcher in examination conditions. The respondents were provided with a pen and an envelope in which to seal their answers and a post-box was used for collection to maintain confidentiality and anonymity. The questionnaires were in both the English and Nepali languages.

Testing of sexual health knowledge

Section 2 of the questionnaire explored young people's knowledge of sexual health matters through the use of 16 true/false statements. The statements fell into four categories; reproductive health, STIs and HIV/AIDS, myths and contraception.

The five statements in the reproductive health category were "It is possible for a women to get pregnant before she has her first period", "There are times in a woman's menstrual cycle when she has a greater chance of becoming pregnant", "A women will not get pregnant if she has sex standing up", "Sexual intercourse whilst pregnant harms the foetus", and "A girl's hymen doesn't tear without sexual intercourse".

The five statements categorized as STIs and HIV/AIDS were "If used properly condoms can protect against HIV transmission", "A person who looks strong and healthy can have HIV", "A person can get AIDS through mosquito, flea and bedbug bites", "There are diseases caught by having sex that can cause a woman to be unable to have a baby" and "A person with an STI can sometimes show no symptoms".

Two statements featured in the mythical grouping, "Masturbation causes serious damage to health" and "A man needs to have sex regularly to maintain his masculinity". Finally, four statements were grouped under the heading of contraception: "The contraceptive pill works just as well even if the women has been sick or had diarrhoea", "Men can have a contraceptive injection (birth control injection) every couple of months to prevent getting a woman pregnant", "Condoms can be used more than once" and "Condoms should not be removed from the penis whilst it is still stiff/hard".

Analytic techniques

The responses of the young men and women to each of the individual 16 knowledge statements were examined and differences between the two sexes identified. Those giving a response of "don't know" were not excluded from the analyses but coded as giving an incorrect answer. Each respondent was allocated four knowledge scores dependent on how many questions they correctly answered in each of the categories, a score of 0 for every incorrect answer, and of 1 for each correct one.

Binary logistic regressions, one for males and one for females, were then fitted to the data to identify the significant factors predictive of correct knowledge.[4] The models were built using both forward and backward conditional stepwise selection procedures; factors were added below the 5 per cent significance level and removed once they became insignificant above that level. Interactions between the variables were also tested for.

Results

Description of the sample

The six educational sites yielded a total of 1,059 completed questionnaires (88 per cent completion rate), 55 per cent of which were

returned by young men. Selected demographic characteristics of the sample
are displayed in table 1. The results displayed in table 2 illustrate the vast
differentials in access to modern amenities experienced by the respondents in
the purposively selected three districts (a consequence of the sampling
strategy employed). In Dhading, no respondents reported having electricity in
their homes, compared with 53 and almost 100 per cent of respondents in
Morang and Lalitpur respectively. Table 2 also highlights the differences
between the three districts in the educational status of pupils' parents. In both
Dhading and Morang, approximately two thirds of mothers were illiterate and,
among women who had received some schooling, very few had attended
beyond primary school. In Lalitpur, though, just over 40 per cent of mothers
had continued education after obtaining their school leaving certificates
(SLC). Among fathers, education attainment was at a similar low level in
Dhading and Morang, whereas in Lalitpur a much greater proportion of fathers
had attained a qualification beyond SLC.

Table 1. Percentage distribution of respondents by selected demographic characteristics

Variable	Grouping	Percentage	N
Sex	Male	54.8	580
	Female	45.2	479
School class	8	11.1	118
	9	52.6	557
	10	36.3	384
Age	14 and under	16.6	176
	15	27.3	289
	16	32.7	346
	17	12.6	133
	18 and above	10.9	115
District	Dhading	17.3	183
	Morang	31.4	333
	Lalitpur	51.3	543
Ethnicity	Brahmin/Chhetri	42.6	451
	Newar	23.5	249
	Rai/Limbu/Sunuwar	10.7	113
	Others	23.2	246
Religion	Hindu	88.7	939
	Buddhist	7.4	78
	Others	2.8	30
	No religion	1.1	12

**Table 2. Percentage distribution of respondents
by selected socio-economic educational indicators**

Indicators	Dhading	Morang	Lalitpur
Socio-economic:			
Drinking water	91.3	91.9	96.1
Electricity	0.0	52.6	99.6
Radio	89.1	62.5	98.9
Freezer	0.0	9.3	76.2
Motorbike	0.0	8.4	52.5
Car	0.0	1.8	22.8
Telephone	0.0	3.9	80.7
Computer	0.0	1.5	47.1
Mother's education:			
Illiterate	66.7	67.6	23.9
Informal	19.7	11.1	7.0
Primary	9.3	14.7	6.3
Some secondary	1.6	5.1	5.3
SLC	0.5	1.5	16.2
Above SLC	2.2	0.0	41.3
Father's education:			
Illiterate	33.3	33.3	9.0
Informal	18.6	9.3	6.8
Primary	27.9	28.2	8.5
Some secondary	7.7	15.0	3.7
SLC	4.9	9.6	7.9
Above SLC	7.7	4.5	64.1

Sources of information

All respondents were asked in the questionnaire who or what were their main sources of information regarding reproductive health (i.e., reproductive system, menstruation, pregnancy, contraception) and HIV/AIDS and other STIs. As illustrated in table 3, the most important sources of information for young people concerning general reproductive health issues were teachers, books, radio and television. Roughly half of the respondents also reported friends of the same sex and health workers as important sources, and young women frequently cited their mother and sister(s) as key resources for reproductive health knowledge.

The main difference found between young people's sources of information concerning reproductive health and STIs and HIV/AIDS was the role of the

**Table 3. Percentage of young men and women reporting various sources
of information regarding reproductive health
(reproductive system, menstruation, pregnancy, contraception)**

Indicators	Male	Female	
Mother	15.7	61.9	***
Father	18.8	12.3	*
Brother(s)	16.0	8.4	***
Sister(s)	6.8	40.7	***
Other family members	13.8	17.8	
Grandparents	9.0	15.0	*
Friends of the same sex	49.2	54.0	
Friends of the opposite sex	12.7	7.9	*
Teachers	79.4	79.5	
Health workers	49.7	50.0	
Television	50.6	55.8	
Cinema	34.1	31.5	
Radio	66.5	64.6	
Books/magazines	65.4	68.2	

*p<0.05   **p<0.01   ***p<0.000

immediate family (see tables 3 and 4). Although mothers of young women appeared
to be a central source regarding reproductive health knowledge, they did not appear to
play such an important role in the provision of information on HIV/AIDs and STIs,
for which fathers seemed to perform a somewhat increased role.

Variations between the three districts in young people's sources were
investigated, with a number of significant differences being found. Young people
whose homes were supplied with electricity were more likely to cite radio and
television as major sources, as would be expected. Further, young women in
Lalitpur were significantly more likely to report their mothers as a source of
information regarding reproductive health issues (69 per cent) than their
counterparts in the other two districts (Dhading: 60 per cent, Morang: 44 per cent);
possibly owing in part to the concentration of more highly educated mothers in
Lalitpur district.

Delivery of sex education in school

Section four of the questionnaire focused on pupils' experiences of the
sex and sexuality education they had received at school. To monitor which
subjects were actually being covered during sex education classes, the pupils were
presented with a list of 11 topics and asked if they had received instruction on each.[5]

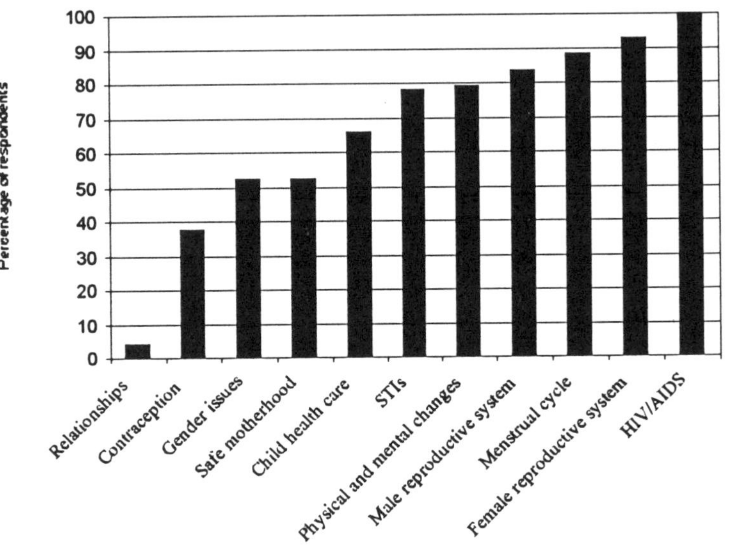

As shown in the figure over three quarters of the pupils in class 10 said they had definitely received instruction about the physical and mental changes which occur during puberty, the reproductive systems of both men and women, the menstrual cycle, HIV/AIDS and STIs. However, just over a third reported having been taught how to protect themselves from pregnancy (contraception) and under five per cent reported having been taught about relationships.

As expected, satisfaction with the issues covered increased significantly as pupils progressed through the school system. Only 15 per cent of pupils sampled in class 8 felt that their health education classes had covered all the sexual health issues they wanted to know about, compared with 28 per cent in class 9 and 40 per cent in class 10. Furthermore, variation was evident between the pupils in each of the six schools. In class 10, students' satisfaction in the different schools ranged from a high of 51 to a low of 30 per cent.

Table 4. Percentage of young men and women reporting various sources of information regarding STIs and HIV/AIDS

Indicators	Male	Female	
Mother	8.7	29.9	***
Father	11.9	21.4	***
Brother(s)	17.0	11.3	*
Sister(s)	7.1	32.3	***
Other family members	15.6	19.2	
Grandparents	7.3	13.7	*
Friends of the same sex	46.1	44.1	
Friends of the opposite sex	14.6	8.6	*
Teachers	83.1	77.4	*
Health workers	55.0	56.7	
Television	58.6	62.7	
Cinema	42.9	41.4	
Radio	69.9	68.4	
Books/magazines	73.8	69.0	

$*p<0.05$ $**p<0.01$ $***p<0.000$

Level of knowledge

Table 5 displays the proportion of young men and women who responded correctly to the 16 true/false statements. It is clear that overall knowledge regarding many of the sexual health issues is relatively low; however, young men appeared to be more informed than their female counterparts, displaying significantly greater knowledge in half of the statements.

The notion that "having sexual intercourse whilst pregnant can harm the foetus" was believed by 95 per cent of both young men and women, almost 70 per cent of young women and 60 per cent of young men believed that "masturbation can cause serious damage to ones' health", a third of young people were aware that STIs can be asymptomatic and only 37 and 20 per cent of young men and women respectively correctly knew that condoms need to be removed from the penis while it is still hard.

Greatest knowledge existed with regard to HIV/AIDS. For example, 73 per cent of men and 60 per cent of women correctly knew that condoms could be used to protect against HIV infection and 71 and 73 per cent of young men and women respectively were aware that "individuals carrying the infection can look strong and healthy".

Table 5. Percentage of respondents correctly responding to each true/false knowledge statement

Knowledge statement		Male	Female	
Reproductive health				
There is the possibility that a woman can get pregnant before she has had her first period	True	7.2	4.4	*
A woman will not get pregnant if she has sex standing up	False	21.0	14.4	*
There are times during a women's menstrual cycle when she has a greater chance of becoming pregnant if she has sex	True	50.7	39.5	***
A girl's hymen doesn't tear without sexual intercourse	False	36.0	39.5	
Sexual intercourse whilst pregnant harms the foetus	False	5.0	5.0	
STIs and HIV/AIDS				
If used properly condoms can protect against HIV transmission	True	73.4	60.1	***
There are diseases caught by having sex that can cause a woman to be unable to have a baby	True	58.8	53.4	
A person who looks strong and healthy can have HIV	True	71	72.7	
A person can get AIDS through mosquito, flea or bedbug bites	False	41.9	45.1	
A person with an STI can sometimes show no symptoms	True	31.7	36.3	
Myths				
Masturbation causes serious damage to health	False	40.7	30.5	**
A man needs to have sex regularly to maintain his masculinity	False	39	43.2	
Contraception				
The contraceptive pill works just as well even if the women has been sick or had diarrhoea	False	22.4	23.2	
Men can have a contraceptive injection (birth control injection) every couple of months to prevent getting a woman pregnant	False	27.9	20.0	**
Condoms can be used more than once	False	57.8	47.6	**
Condoms should not be removed from the penis while it is still hard/stiff	False	37.1	20.0	***

*p<0.05   **p<0.01   ***p<0.000

School site	Reproductive health (0-5)	STIs and HIV/AIDs (0-5)	Myths (0-2)	Contraception (0-4)
Males				
Dhading (1)	0.77	1.99	0.95	1.59
Morang (1)	1.39	2.84	0.66	1.34
Morang (2)	1.22	2.61	0.63	1.54
Lalitpur (1)	1.30	3.41	0.90	1.34
Lalitpur (2)	1.11	2.26	0.82	1.56
Lalitpur (3)	1.38	3.32	0.89	1.45
Sig	0.000	0.000	0.001	0.317
Females				
Dhading (1)	0.71	1.71	0.86	1.06
Morang (1)	1.36	2.12	0.51	1.05
Morang (2)	1.53	2.47	0.43	1.40
Lalitpur (1)	0.96	3.44	0.79	1.07
Lalitpur (2)	0.97	1.79	0.79	1.24
Lalitpur (3)	1.09	3.44	0.78	1.09
Sig	0.000	0.000	0.003	0.556

Table 6 displays the school-level mean scores for both men and women in each of the four knowledge categories. As shown, significant differences in knowledge between the six sites were apparent for all topics except that of contraceptive knowledge.

The maximum possible knowledge score in the reproductive health category was 5. No pupil received full marks and only eight pupils correctly answered four out of the five questions; 64 per cent of young men and 73 per cent of women scored less than two. General knowledge regarding contraception was also found to be low, with only 3 and 2 per cent of men and women, respectively, correctly answering all four questions as compared with 19 and 34 per cent respectively not getting any of the answers correct. More encouraging were the scores for STI and HIV/AIDS knowledge. Overall, 9 per cent of men and women correctly answered all five questions and only 15 per cent of men and 20 per cent of women scored less than two.

Determinants of knowledge

It would appear that success, to a certain degree, has been achieved in the delivery of health messages concerning HIV/AIDS, the statements "individuals with HIV/AIDS can look strong and healthy" and "when used properly condoms can protect against HIV" (the two highest-scoring statements) were therefore selected as dependent variables in the logistic regressions performed to identify factors associated with increased knowledge.

When used properly condoms can protect against HIV

Factors found to be predictive of young people's knowledge concerning the use of condoms to protect against HIV are displayed in table 7. As shown, young men who live in Morang have a little over seven times the odds of knowing that condoms protect against HIV as young men who live in Dhading district; likewise, young men in Lalitpur have 1.8 times the odds. Similar findings are evident among the young women, where odds are increased by about 21 and 6 times in Morang and Lalitpur, respectively. As a young person progresses through the school system, knowledge is found to increase significantly. Young men and women in class 10 are 3.1 and over 10 times, respectively, as likely to have correct knowledge about condoms than their peers in class 8, after controlling for all other factors. School type also appears to impact on levels of knowledge. Students attending the privately run school were found to have up to 3 times the odds of correct knowledge as similar students attending State-run establishments.

Other factors found to be significant in the male model included the cited sources of information regarding HIV and topics covered during sex education classes delivered at school. As illustrated in table 7, young men who reported their brothers, television and magazines/books as main sources of information on HIV/AIDS were roughly 2 to 3 times as likely in each case to correctly know that condoms can protect against HIV if used properly as those who did not cite each as sources. Finally, young men who had received basic sex education at school (the physical and mental changes that occur at puberty, the male reproductive system and safe motherhood) had significantly greater odds of knowledge than those who had not attended classes, after all other factors had been controlled for.

Additional significant knowledge predictors in the female model included religion, father's educational level, sex education received at school, and television and books as main sources of HIV/AIDS information.

Table 7. Odds ratios from logistic regression analyses predicting the effects of various characteristics on the likelihood of correct knowledge

Characteristic		Odds ratio
Men		
District	Dhading	1.00
	Morang	7.42 ***
	Lalitpur	1.79
Class	8	1.00
	9	1.87
	10	3.14 **
Source of HIV information	Brother	3.05 *
	Television	2.33 **
	Books/magazines	2.29 **
Sex education received	Physical and mental changes	2.04 *
	Male reproductive system	2.57 **
	Safe motherhood	2.44 **
Type of school	Public	1.00
	Private	2.47 *
Constant		0.03
Df		11
-2 Log likelihood		469.70
Women		
District	Dhading	1.00
	Morang	21.26 ***
	Lalitpur	5.82 ***
Class	8	1.00
	9	5.79 **
	10	10.19 **
Religion	Non-Hindu	1.00
	Hindu	0.33 *
Father's education	Illiterate	1.00
	Primary/informal	2.92 *
	Secondary/SLC	1.32
	Above SLC	3.98 **
Source of HIV information	Television	1.98 *
	Books/magazines	3.49 ***
Sex education received	Physical and mental changes	5.39 ***
	The menstrual cycle	0.32 *
Type of school	Public	1.00
	Private	2.94 *
Constant		0.007 ***
Df		13
-2 Log likelihood		355.54

*p<0.05   **p<0.01   ***p<0.000

Young women who practised Hinduism were significantly less likely to respond with the correct answer and, after controlling for all other factors, young women with more educated fathers were more likely to respond correctly. For example, women whose fathers were educated above SLC level had almost 4 times the odds of being correct as those with illiterate fathers.

The sources of information which were found to significantly impact on knowledge among young women concerning the use of condoms as a protection against HIV included television and magazines/books, which increased the odds by 2.0 and 3.5 times respectively. As with young men, young women who reported basic sex education teaching at school (physical and mental changes at puberty) were significantly more likely to have correct knowledge; however, after controlling for all other factors, young women who had received teaching on the menstrual cycle were 68 per cent less likely to respond correctly (although this finding was only just significant at the 5 per cent level).

People who have HIV/AIDS can look strong and healthy

Factors found to be predictive of young men's and women's knowledge concerning the appearance of individuals infected with HIV are displayed in table 8.

Father's level of education appeared to be a significant predictor of correct knowledge among the young men sampled. For example, young men whose fathers were educated to degree standard had 2.3 times the odds of providing a correct response as young men who had illiterate fathers. Furthermore, young men who reported books and television as a main source of information regarding HIV/AIDS had roughly twice the odds of knowing that people infected with HIV can look strong and healthy as those not accessing such sources. Young men who rely on teachers as an informative source were, however, found to be significantly less likely to respond correctly.

Having received basic sex education at school (physical and mental changes during puberty and the male reproductive system) was also found to be significantly associated with odds of correct knowledge; however, unlike the previous model, receiving safe motherhood education at school this time decreased the odds by 43 per cent, after controlling for all other factors.

Having received basic sex education at school (physical and mental changes during puberty and the male reproductive system) was also found to be significantly associated with odds of correct knowledge; however, unlike the previous model, receiving safe motherhood education at school this time decreased the odds by 43 per cent, after controlling for all other factors.

Table 8. Odds ratios from logistic regression analyses predicting the effects of various characteristics on the likelihood of correct knowledge regarding the healthy appearance of individuals infected with HIV

Characteristics		Odds ratio	
Men			
Father's education	Illiterate	1.00	
	Primary/informal	0.80	
	Secondary/SLC	2.80	**
	Above SLC	2.31	**
Source of HIV information	Teachers	0.55	*
	Television	2.22	**
	Books/magazines	2.39	***
Sex education received	Physical and mental changes	1.71	*
	Male reproductive system	2.51	**
	Safe motherhood	0.57	**
Constant		0.50	
Df		9	
-2 Log likelihood		602.15	
Women			
Mother's education	Illiterate	1.00	
	Primary/informal	1.06	
	Secondary/SLC	5.49	**
	Above SLC	2.16	(10%)
Source of HIV information	Books/magazines	2.43	***
Sex education received	Male reproductive system	1.89	*
	Relationships	4.13	*
Number of amenities /	0-2	1.00	
household assets	3-5	0.92	
	6-7	2.90	**
	8-10	1.90	(10%)
Constant		0.44	
Df		9	
-2 Log likelihood		458.13	

*p<0.05   ** p<0.01 ***p<0.000

Among the young women, mothers' education appeared to be a good predictor of knowledge; young women whose mothers had completed secondary education or higher had significantly raised odds of correct knowledge. The use of written literature as a source of HIV/AIDS information provided young women with significantly increased knowledge, and young women who reported receiving some basic sex education including the teaching of the male reproductive system and the role of relationships were roughly 2 and 4 times as likely to know that HIV-infected individuals can look healthy as similar young women not receiving such instruction. Finally, level of social-economic deprivation, as measured by the number of amenities in the household, significantly impacted on the likelihood that a young woman knew that people with HIV can look strong and healthy, with young women living in more affluent households displaying greater awareness.

Discussion

In the context of a global decline in age of sexual maturation and rising age of marriage, the window of opportunity for young people to engage in premarital sexual relations is opening. Social taboos and inhibitions have in the past limited the study of Nepalese young people's sexual knowledge, attitudes and behaviour; however, with the advent of HIV/AIDS and increasing prevalence of STIs there has been a realization of the need to provide young people with information and skills to reduce their vulnerability to negative sexual health outcomes.

The results presented here are from a sex and sexuality education survey distributed among young people at secondary school. It forms part of a much larger study looking at the barriers and opportunities to developing a more comprehensive sex education curriculum. It is recognized that the analyses are based on a relatively small proportion of young people in Nepal and include only those attending school. Also, the purposive sampling techniques employed mean that the final respondent sample is not truly representative of all young people in school classes 8, 9 and 10. Nevertheless, the results highlight several key issues which merit further attention and have a direct bearing on health promotion and school curriculum development activities.

With regard to young people's sources of information about sexual health issues, the results from this study clearly show that schools play an important role in informing young people about sexual health matters. However, on examination of the topics that are being covered in class, it is apparent that the more easily taught, less challenging, factual and biological issues are fairly consistently being covered, whereas the broader issues such as feelings and relationships are often being overlooked. Although it is crucial that young people be given the basic facts on such things as the male and female reproductive systems, the menstrual cycle, HIV/AIDS and methods of contraception, unless these are provided in conjunction with the skills training to enable young people to communicate their wishes and desires effectively, it is unlikely that the knowledge gained will lead to effective behaviour change.

This study found in-depth knowledge regarding many sexual health issues to be low among both young men and young women in Nepal, with the exception of particular knowledge concerning HIV/AIDS. Although young men appear to be better informed than young women, myths about masturbation and virility remain widespread and detailed knowledge regarding contraception remains sparse.

The results of the modelling, which attempts to identify factors predictive of HIV/AIDS knowledge, show that awareness regarding the use of condoms to avoid exposure to HIV infection improves as pupils move up through the school classes; however, clear disparities are evident between the districts and schools sampled. Young people living in the most remote district, Dhading, with little access to modern media, have significantly reduced levels of knowledge, compared with young people living in the more developed districts of Morang and Lalitpur, after controlling for all other factors. Furthermore, pupils, and in particular female students, in Morang district, appeared to be better informed than their counterparts in Lalitpur. This unexpected outcome, given the relative levels of social deprivation and modernization in the two districts, could possibly be explained by the presence of a Healthy Schools Programme in Morang, run by PLAN International.[6] Although the initiative is not being implemented in the specific schools included in this particular study, the information that is being provided by the programme could possibly be filtering into the wider community and thereby increasing overall knowledge.

Parental education, rather than district of residence, was found to be a much greater predictor of knowledge regarding the healthy appearance of individuals infected with HIV. This finding could purely be a reflection of the differential levels of development in the three regions; alternatively, it might be that more educated parents, having greater awareness of the impact that HIV can have on an individual's health, subsequently transfer correct knowledge to their children.

In all the models, the detrimental effect of social deprivation on young people's level of knowledge is highly evident along with the positive impact that exposure to visual media messages and access to informative sources of literature can have. In every instance, young people who cite television and magazines/books as main sources of information on HIV have substantially increased odds of correct knowledge. Finally, but by no means least, young people who have received basic sex education at school are, in general, better informed as a result, even after controlling for all other factors including age, district, social deprivation and exposure to media.

Although this research, on which further work is required, leaves a number of key questions unanswered, it is clear that if the desired shift in behaviour to reduce HIV/AIDS and STI prevalence and the number of unwanted pregnancies is to be achieved, we need to take a multifarious approach to delivering knowledge to tackle the issues. Appropriately designed and relevant educational activities need to be targeted, not only at young people, but also at the parents and elderly persons from whom they seek information and guidance. The results of this study would indicate that media messages delivered via visual means are effective; however, many people in Nepal do not have access to such amenities so alternative means of transferring messages need to be explored. Since many people are also illiterate, this is not a simple task.

Although Nepal has incorporated sex and sexuality education into its national curriculum, it is still very much in its infancy and requires further monitoring and evaluation. Nevertheless, given the relatively short period of time that the programme has been running, the results presented here clearly show the potential that schools have to contribute to improved learning about sexual and reproductive health matters. Detailed and comprehensive knowledge among many young people, and in particular young women, appears to be remain low, emphasizing the need for further curriculum and teacher training material development with a shift away from superficial biological coverage towards a more inclusive programme.

Acknowledgements

The authors would like to thank all the hard-pressed teaching staff who agreed to distribute the questionnaires; all the young people who diligently completed the questionnaire; all the staff at SOLID Nepal for successfully completing the project under such unstable working conditions; Mahesh Puri and Govinda Dahal, who commented on earlier drafts; and DFID for funding the study.

Endnotes

1. Age and sex distribution unspecified.

2. Classes are organized by level of ability not by age; however, ages of the sample ranged from a low of 12 to a high of 22 with 87 per cent aged between 14 and 17 years.

3. All schools, whether government-run or private, are obliged to cover the same curriculum.

4. Factors tested in the model included: district, school site and type, age, class, ethnicity/caste, religion, importance of religion, sources of HIV/AIDS information, topics covered during school sex education classes, highest educational level of mother and father, and level of socio-economic deprivation.

5. Each of these 11 topics are listed in the curriculum handbook.

6. A child-focused, non-profit developmental organization aiding deprived children in developing countries.

References

Aryal, R. H. and D. Nichols (2002). *Birth Planning among Urban Youth in Nepal: Awareness, Knowledge, Perceptions and Practice*, NAYA report series No. 13 (Kathmandu, Family Health International).

Dahal, G. P. (1999). "An insight on the recommendations of the ICPD Programme of Action: emerging challenges to implement reproductive health policy in Nepal", *FPAN Journal of Reproductive Health*, vol. 1, No. 1, pp. 32-44.

Furber, A. S., J. N. Newell and M.M. Lubben (2002). "A systematic review of current knowledge of HIV epidemiology and of sexual behaviour in Nepal", *Tropical Medicine and International Health*, vol. 7, No. 2, pp. 140-148.

Grunseit, A. and others (1997). "Sexuality education and young people's sexual behavior: a review of studies", *Journal of Adolescent Research*, vol. 12, No. 4, pp. 421-453.

Khanal, H. (1999). "Adolescent reproductive health in Nepal", *FPAN Journal of Reproductive Health*, vol. 1, No. 1, pp. 45-53.

Kirby, D. (2001). *Emerging Answers: Research Findings on Programs to Reduce Teen Pregnancy* (Washington, National Campaign to Prevent Teenage Pregnancy).

Limbu, R. (2001). "Nepal: let's talk about sex", Inter Press Service, 12 October (*<www.aegis.com/news/ips/2001/IP011005.html>*).

Mehta, S. (1998). Responsible Sexual and Reproductive Health Behaviour among Adolescents (United Nations Population Fund).

Nepal (1998). Ministry of Education, Department of Education (<*www.nepallink.com/nepal/lifestyle/education.php3*>).

Nepal Demographic and Health Survey (NDHS) (1996). Demographic and Health Surveys STATcomplier [online]. Measure DHS+. Available from: <*http://www.measuredhs.com*>.

___________ (2001). Demographic and Health Surveys STAT complier [online]. Measure DHS+. Available from: <*http://www.measuredhs.com*>.

Neupane, S. and D. Nichols (2002). *HIV/AIDS and Other Sexually Transmitted Infections in Nepal: Knowledge and Beliefs among Urban Youth*, NAYA report series No. 14 (Kathmandu, Family Health International).

Pradhan, A., and others (1997). *Nepal Family Health Survey 1996* (Kathmandu and Calverton, Maryland, Ministry of Health of Nepal, New ERA and Macro International Inc.).

Prasai, D. P. (1999). "Effectiveness of sexuality education program in Palpa district of Nepal", *FPAN Journal of Reproductive Health*, vol. 1, No. 1, pp. 6-12.

Puri, M. (2002). *Sexual Risk Behaviour and Risk Perception of Unwanted Pregnancy and Sexually Transmitted Infection among Young Factory Workers in Nepal* (Kathmandu, Centre for Research on Environment Health and Population Activities).

Tamang, A., and others (2001). "Sexual behaviour and risk perceptions among young men in border towns of Nepal", *Asia-Pacific Population Journal*, vol. 16, No. 2, June 2001, pp. 195-210.

UNFPA (1996). *Reproductive Tract Infections including STDs and HIV/AIDS in Nepal* (Kathmandu, UNFPA).

Reproductive Health including Family Planning

*The integration of family planning into expanded
reproductive health programmes that provide women and men
with choice in planning their reproductive lives, while still incomplete,
has not led to reversals in fertility decline*

By Philip Guest

Despite occasional efforts to reverse the consensus articulated in the Programme of Action of the International Conference on Population and Development (ICPD), for almost a decade the recommendations contained in this Programme of Action have provided the guiding framework for expanding and reorienting reproductive health programmes in the Asian and Pacific region. Reproductive health in the above-mentioned Programme is defined as "a state of complete physical, mental and social well-being and not merely the absence of disease or infirmity, in all matters relating to the reproductive system and to its functions and processes" (para. 7.2). Reproductive health services are viewed as a basic right through which women and men can express their reproductive choices.

The High-level Meeting to Review the Implementation of the Programme of Action of the International Conference on Population and Development and the Bali Declaration on Population and Sustainable Development and to Make Recommendations for Further Action, which was held at Bangkok in 1998, highlighted the progress that many countries in the region had made in integrating family planning with other reproductive health services and improving the quality of care provided in their family planning programmes. However, the Meeting also noted that major obstacles remained in implementing the recommendations contained in the Programme of Action. Some of the obstacles related to the capacity of the service system to provide expanded services, some to cultural barriers, particularly those related to gender inequality, that limited the reproductive health options of women and some to weak government commitment. The Meeting made a number of recommendations that were designed to manifest further commitment to the ICPD goals and remove obstacles to attaining the goals (ESCAP 1998).

In Asia, there has been continuing debate over the role of national family planning programmes in reproductive health programmes. While national family programmes have undoubtedly contributed to rapidly declining fertility in many Asian countries through allowing couples to achieve their desired family size, the very success of the programmes has resulted in a diminishing interest in using public moneys to fund them. However, the changes in orientation towards family planning and reproductive health that have existed since the late 1980s and that were legitimated by ICPD have provided family planning programmes with new roles and a new purpose.

In this paper several issues are examined. In the first section of the paper, the author summarizes selected aspects of family planning programmes in the region. In the second section, the linkages between family planning and other aspects of reproductive health are examined. The third section of the paper focuses on quality-of-care issues related to reproductive health, while in the final section of the paper new roles for reproductive health programmes are examined.

Family planning programmes in the Asian and Pacific region

Caldwell and others (2002: 10) state that the twenty-first century started with "the greatest number of national family planning programs in position that had ever existed". Asian countries have been leaders in the establishment of family planning programmes and despite the remarkable fertility declines that occurred in most of East and South-East Asia over the preceding decades, the number of programmes continues to grow rather than diminish.

Table 1. Percentage of currently married women aged 15-49 using contraceptives by type of method: nine selected populous countries

Country and year	Percentage using contraceptive method			
	Any method	Sterilization	Any modern temporary method	Any traditional method
China, 1997	84	41	42	1
India, 1998/99	48	36	7	5
Indonesia, 1997	57	3	51	3
Pakistan, 1995/95	18	5	8	5
Bangladesh, 1999/2000	54	7	36	10
Viet Nam, 1994	65	4	39	21
Philippines, 1998	47	10	18	18
Iran (Islamic Republic of), 1992	65	9	37	20
Thailand, 1993	74	23	50	2

Source: East-West Center (2002).

For the entire Asian region, by the year 2000 the total fertility rate (TFR) had dropped to levels that are intermediate between 2 and 3. Well over one half of currently married women in reproductive ages were using contraception, and population growth had slowed appreciably. These changes have been facilitated by the presence of national family planning programmes in most of the countries of the region. There remains, however, significant diversity in the levels and methods of contraceptive use among countries in the region.

In table 1, the contraceptive prevalence rates for nine populous countries in Asia are shown. In several of the countries approximately two thirds or more of currently married reproductive-aged women were using contraceptives. For Pakistan the contraceptive prevalence rate was below 20 per cent. In India there is a particularly high reliance on sterilization, while in countries such as Indonesia and Viet Nam sterilization comprises a small proportion of methods used. Meanwhile, in other countries, traditional methods, primarily the calendar method and withdrawal, contribute a large proportion to overall levels of contraceptive use.

Many of the differences among countries in the levels of contraceptive use and contraceptive method mix can be linked to the evolution of national family planning programmes in the region. Jones and Leete (2002: 117) characterize the 1970s as the "heyday of family planning programmes in Asia." It was during this decade that many countries established their family planning programmes in a context of growing international and domestic concern over the need to reduce fertility. International funding was available for family planning programmes, and a focus on the measurable outcome of achieving targeted lower levels of population growth helped motivate programmes.

The emphasis on achieving fertility decline resulted in family planning programmes in several countries, particularly in South Asia, focusing on permanent methods. Pakistan, a country with a long-established family planning programme, has had difficulty in achieving political support and commitment and this is reflected in low levels of use, and a relatively high proportion of use consisting of non-modern methods. The Philippines is another country where political commitment to family planning has waxed and waned and where the use of non-modern methods is high. In Viet Nam, political commitment to family planning has not been a problem. However, despite recent efforts to broaden contraceptive choice and improve quality of care, it appears that concerns about the quality of services have contributed to relatively high levels of use of non-modern contraceptives.

In many countries with newly established programmes, success was quick in coming. In Thailand, TFR, which had already been declining before the national family planning programme commenced in 1970, declined from over 6 during the latter half of the 1960s to below 4 by the end of the 1970s. Although fertility decline in Thailand has been ascribed to a number of factors (Knodel and others 1987), the flexible approach of the family planning programme and its willingness to respond to interventions successfully piloted by an active non-governmental organizational (NGO) community, helped to facilitate the decline.

Harbison and Robinson (2002) argue that the main reason for the success of family planning programmes in reducing fertility was that they were able to convince the public of the benefits of a small family. In turn, other societal forces contributing to the ideational change favouring fewer children helped to contribute to some family planning programmes being considered as very successful. This argument implies that where family programmes have been able to cater for the emerging needs of women for effective contraception, and where they have in some way been able to help to legitimize those needs, programmes have been successful in attaining the policy objective of lower fertility. The extent to which reproductive health programmes, including family planning, can address the reproductive health needs of women and men will continue to determine their success.

The role of family planning in reproductive health

The centrality of family planning to reproductive health in the post-Cairo era has been reiterated in several international population forums (see Khan and others 1998). The provision of quality family planning services provides couples with the ability to choose the timing and number of children they will have. Family planning services undertaken in isolation from other aspects of reproductive health weaken the commitment to providing couples, and particularly women, with the full range of reproductive health services that they require to lead healthy lives. Family planning is a crucial aspect of services since it provides couples with the ability to make choices about their reproductive goals and it is these choices that have implications for health. In much of the region, family planning programmes are the primary organizational structure for implementing policies designed to affect non-contraceptive aspects of reproductive health, so the role of family planning programmes must be recognized and adapted to help to solve reproductive health concerns. Finally, and a fact not recognized by many family planning programmes, women themselves make a link between family planning and their reproductive health. Often this is in terms of the perceived health risk that they feel they will be exposed to if they adopt family planning.

Family planning and mortality reduction

The links between family planning and infant and child mortality are now well established, even if the magnitude of the effect continues to be debated. Over the past decade a number of studies in several Asian countries have demonstrated how the use of contraception, resulting in few children and longer spacing between children, has contributed to improved maternal and child health (see Greenspan 1993; Luther and others 1999; Miller and others 1992; Popkin and others 1993). There are a series of interrelated factors that affect the probability of an infant dying. The shorter the interval between births, the higher the parity of the child, and births occurring at the extremes of a woman's reproductive career are all associated with higher probabilities of infant deaths. Estimates of the differentials in mortality associated with each of these effects give some indication of the potential for infant mortality decline if contraception was more widely used to space or limit fertility.   For example, probabilities of death are up to 2.5 times higher where the birth interval is less than 2 years compared with birth intervals of more than 2 years; the probability of death of an infant of parity 7 or more can be up to 2 times higher than for parities 1 to 3, and women giving birth from age 18 to 34 may be up to 50 per cent less likely to have their infant die compared with mothers aged less than 18, and about 25 per cent less likely compared with mothers aged 35 and over.

Many of the issues that relate infant and child mortality to fertility can also be applied to maternal mortality.   Without there being any changes in socio-economic conditions or access to health services, a reduction in fertility would result in a reduction in maternal mortality. This would occur in an absolute sense, with the number of mothers dying declining, and in a relative sense, with the probability of maternal death associated with each birth declining. This latter effect would occur because fertility decline results in a reduction of births occurring to high-risk groups. Based on data from the Matlab in Bangladesh, Fortney (1987) demonstrates that if births at ages of mothers less than 20 and greater than 39 and births of parities greater than 5 were eliminated, the maternal mortality ratio would decrease by 25 per cent while the number of women dying in the age group 15 to 49 would decrease by 56 per cent.

International commitment to Safe Motherhood has increased over the last decade, primarily as a result of the ICPD Programme of Action. There is now a much better appreciation of what are priority interventions and how and where these interventions might be integrated into family planning programmes (Berer and Ravindran 1999).

The indirect effects of family planning on improved morbidity and mortality of mothers and children are harder to document than the direct effects but are probably equally strong. At the societal level, fertility decline can reduce the overall levels of dependency and hence increase the per capita level of resources available for investment in health services for the dependent population. This can also occur at the household level: small families have greater wealth than larger families and hence can devote more resources to improving the health of family members. Access to family planning programmes can also be an entry point for women into the wider health system. This can lead to better health for women and their families.

A contentious issue that many family planning programmes prefer to avoid is the issue of abortion. Ahman and Shah (2002) estimate that in the year 2000, there were 19 million unsafe abortions and of these, over 50 per cent (10.5 million) occurred in Asia. Unsafe abortion is a major contributor to maternal mortality, with annually over 80,000 deaths of women, the vast majority in developing countries, attributed to unsafe abortions (WHO 1998). The presence of a high level of abortion is one indication of difficulties of women obtaining access to appropriate methods of effective contraception. In many fertility transitions, initial declines in fertility were associated with increases in the incidence of induced abortion. As effective contraception became available, the level of abortion was reduced. In many developing societies, abortion-related deaths are most likely to occur for women in their twenties; therefore, family planning can have a major impact on reducing the risk of maternal mortality at ages where, in the absence of abortion, the risk of maternal mortality is very low. Increases in premarital sexual activity, the difficulty of unmarried women obtaining access to contraception and/or social factors which tend to discourage the use of contraception for the unmarried are also related to increased levels of abortion and attendant mortality risks for young women.

In those areas of the Asian and Pacific region where son preference of children is strong, there continues to be the problems of sex-selective abortions (East-West Center 2002). Bairagi (2001), in a study of the effects of son preference in Bangladesh, notes that the effect of son preference on abortion has increased over time and that if foetal sex identification becomes more widely available, the number of abortions of female foetuses may increase. Other countries in the region where sex- selective abortion has been a concern include China, India and the Republic of Korea. While these countries have combated the problems through legislation banning foetal sex identification, change in the underlying societal values that result in son preference requires more programmatic attention.

Some of the issues not discussed here, but which deserve fuller treatment, are the effects of family planning on other aspects of a family's life. There is a growing body of evidence that families who limit fertility are able to invest more resources in improving the human capital of their children (better health and education) and in increasing the economic resources of the family. Of course these outcomes are not only a result of the adoption of family planning, but can also be seen as a major motivation for the acceptance of family planning. It is notable that the presence of these relationships is most evident in societies in which the fertility transition is well advanced, suggesting that when couples realize the benefits to their family from limiting fertility, they are quick to practise contraception.

Family planning and reproductive morbidities

In the years leading up to ICPD at Cairo in 1994, evidence emerged of the high levels of reproductive tract infections (RTIs) in developing countries. Bang and others (1989) reported high level of both endogenous RTIs and sexually transmitted infections (STIs) in rural India. Other studies in India have also reported high levels of RTIs (Bhatia and Cleland 1995). Similar results have been reported in other Asian countries such as China and Viet Nam (Kaufman and others 1999; Lien and others 2002).

Since Cairo the provision of RTI/STI services have been seen as an important area of integration with family planning services (Walker 1998). In part this is because methods such as the IUD should not be provided unless it has been determined that the client does not suffer from an RTI. Also, women often see symptoms of RTIs as an outcome of their contraceptive use and hence seek assistance from family planning services when they experience possible RTI symptoms such as vaginal discharge.

The ability of family planning clinics in resource-poor settings to effectively diagnose and treat RTIs requires further investigation. Lien and others (2002), based on their study in Viet Nam, argue that investing in establishing and maintaining diagnostic facilities may not be the most efficient use of resources at the local level. Instead, they provide several alternative options that involve more simplified procedures for diagnosis of RTIs. Kaufman and others (1999) came to similar conclusions based on their study in China. What is clear is that any treatment strategy adopted for RTIs within family planning programmes needs to be based on knowledge of the levels and composition of RTIs within each area.

Even in situations where it is not possible to integrate diagnosis and treatment of RTIs into the operations of family planning programme service delivery points, it is possible to include prevention in programmes. For areas where STIs/HIV are a concern, this could include promotion and distribution of condoms, HIV pre- and post-test counselling and referral. For RTIs, education on recognizing RTIs and appropriate care-seeking behaviour could be provided.

Quality of care in reproductive health services

As part of the demographic argument, and also as a recognition of the human rights and dignity of clients, programmes are now stressing the quality of care provided to clients. It has been shown that where a variety of methods are available, where communication between service provider and client is open and two-way and where service providers are well trained, current users are more likely to continue using contraceptives and to use their chosen method of contraception more effectively. The quality of care framework (see Bruce 1990), provides a set of guidelines that programme managers can use to reorient their activities to make them more consistent with the reproductive rights recommendations of the ICPD Programme of Action.

A central component of the Bruce framework is that clients should have a real choice of methods. Ross and others (2002), in a cross-national study, have shown that availability of methods is strongly related to the prevalence of each method and that overall prevalence is related to the overall availability of several methods. Because couples have different contraceptive needs and preferences, and as these needs and preferences vary over their life, a programme should ideally include a range of methods in order to cater for the various inclinations. Where a variety of methods are available to meet the varying needs of clients, one can expect prevalence and client satisfaction to be highest.

Khan, Boon-Ann and Mehta (1998) in their assessment of the quality of care of family planning programmes in the Asian and Pacific region five years after ICPD noted that in many programmes there were a limited number of methods available and that in some programmes where a variety of methods were available, provider biases or method-based incentives reduced choice. While programme managers at the national level have shown clear commitment to broaden effective choice, the understanding of informed choice and indeed the whole concept of quality of care have been shown to be lacking among many providers (Abdullah 1999).

The consequences of a lack of informed choice are low levels of client satisfaction, high levels of contraceptive discontinuation and increased numbers of unplanned pregnancies. Johansson and others (1996), in a study of abortion in two villages in Viet Nam, argue that many abortions were related to the limited choice of contraceptives available in the service delivery system. Essentially the only method available was the IUD and many women who had discontinued IUD use because of side effects became pregnant and resorted to abortion.

Informed choice of methods does not simply mean making all methods available. Programmes need to be able to incorporate the new methods into their service delivery system and clients must fully understand the implications of using each method. The inappropriate inclusion of a method into a service delivery system can have adverse impacts on women's health and increase the risk of an unplanned pregnancy. Hull (1998) describes how in an eastern province of Indonesia a lack of knowledge and skill among providers in the removal of contraceptive implants, combined with a related lack of understanding of clients about when removal should occur or even if it should occur, resulted in many women not having the implants removed at the appropriate time.

The difficulties in instituting real informed choice of contraceptive methods is clearly shown in the case of China. China's family planning programme has operated with strict and clearly defined birth limitation rules and within the context of one main method on, the IUD (see Attané 2002; Winckler 2002). In the years following ICPD, the Government of China has taken steps to relax some aspects of their programme through promoting aspects of quality-of-care, while retaining population regulations. These steps, which were tentative at first, have now quickened and there are quality of care initiatives in many of the numerous counties in China. One pilot project, designed to introduce informed contraceptive choice, commenced in Deqing county of Zhejiang province in 1995. An assessment of the pilot project in 1998 shows that within the confines of a strict and mandatory policy on the number of births allowed, women are being provided with greater choice of methods and that this results in greater satisfaction for them and has also oriented providers to the importance of women's preferences (Gu and others 2002).

A central component of instituting a client-centred approach to reproductive health services, particularly family planning services, is the removal of targets within family planning programmes. The record of abolition of targets in the family planning programmes of countries in the region is very mixed. Of 25 Asian and Pacific countries and areas responding to an ESCAP questionnaire about their reproductive health programmes in the five years after Cairo, 18 said that their programmes had included quantitative targets and only 4 responded that they had removed those targets after Cairo. India was one of the countries that reported removing programme targets (ESCAP 1998). Murthy and others (2002), based on the results of three case studies in various parts of India, found that experiences varied markedly between their three research sites. In all sites some progress towards eliminating targets was achieved, but the extent of change was limited. Significantly, they note that easing targets did not reduce contraceptive levels and may have resulted in increased use of temporary methods. The findings of this study illustrate the difficulties of changing entrenched practices at lower levels of family planning programmes.

However, attempts are being made within the region to change practices not consistent with the quality-of-care approach. For example, Jain and others (2002) report on a pilot project in the Philippines that used information about the needs of clients, expressed by the clients, to design provider work plans and direct service efforts. This new approach replaced an existing system based primarily on demographic and medical criteria. Unfortunately, this example of a client-centred management approach to providing services is the exception rather than the norm.

Other aspects of quality of care also need to be improved in reproductive health programmes in Asia and the Pacific. Schuler and Hossain (1998), for example, argue that there remain major problems or poor interpersonal communication between providers and clients in the Bangladesh national family planning programme. They recommend that institutional norms, policies and incentives have to follow a client-centred approach if these problems are to be overcome. Koenig and others (2000), in a review of studies that have examined the quality of care under the India Family Welfare Programme, suggest that even though some changes in the Indian Family Welfare Programme were made in 1996 and 1997 to accommodate ICPD recommendations, there has been little improvement at the local level. They state that most studies indicate a lack of concern for client needs and preferences, and that poor women are particularly disadvantaged within the programme in obtaining an appropriate quality of care. Although direct evidence is lacking, they state: "poor quality of care likely has contributed to high levels of foregone, delayed, or discontinued practice of contraception and consequently to unwanted pregnancy among current or potential clients" (p. 13).

Overall there has been progress in improving the quality of care provided in reproductive health programmes in the Asian and Pacific region. However, this progress has been hampered by a lack of understanding and appreciation of the importance of client preferences and by service delivery systems that are resistant to change (Abdullah 1999). Change in reproductive health programmes has been most apparent in improvement in the quality of services rather than in terms of quality of care. A similar conclusion is also made by Hardee and others (1999, p. s8), who state that the "reproductive rights aspects of Cairo have received far less attention than the health aspects".

Priority roles for family planning programmes

Much of the region, especially areas of South Asia, remains in a situation where birth rates are high, levels of contraceptive use are low, unmet need for family planning is high and childbirth is accompanied by a high risk of death for both the mother and her new-born infant. In these countries, efforts need to be made to ensure that individuals are provided with the means to achieve their desired family sizes within programmes that provide the highest possible quality of care. In these countries, to the extent practicable, other elements of reproductive health should be integrated with family planning.

There are many other developing countries in the region, however, which have made great strides in increasing contraceptive use, lowering birth rates and improving the health of mothers and children. It is the situation in this latter group of countries, particularly with regard to the roles of family planning programmes, that is focused upon below.

Serving vulnerable groups

What are the roles that the family planning programmes of these countries should play? Should the structure and funding patterns of the programmes change? Should the programmes exist at all? These questions are being faced by a number of family planning programmes in South-East and East Asia. Jones and Leete (2002) argue that there are two priorities for family planning programmes of countries in the region where fertility has fallen below replacement level. The first is to turn over more of the provision of contraceptive and other reproductive health services to the private sector. Potts and others (1999) argue that shortfalls in expected international and domestic resources for reproductive health services require that much more emphasis be placed on commercial family planning services in developing countries. The role of the Government in this situation would be to ensure that the quality of services is maintained at a high standard and that services to those segments of the population that cannot afford to pay for them are maintained.

Ensuring that vulnerable groups have access to affordable reproductive health services in a context where many programmes are attempting to broaden user fees is a priority issue for Governments. In countries where high priority is placed on family planning, such as China, this can mean that family planning services remain free to all through the government family planning services. In other areas of reproductive health, such as maternal care, where user fees are required, there is increasing concern that many poorer women do not have access to services (IHS 2002). Although many couples in China could undoubtedly afford to pay for family planning services, and indeed many urban women do so, there remains a need to subsidize access to the full range of reproductive health services for poorer women.

There are other population groups that for one reason or another do not have access to reproductive health services. Lack of access may result from social barriers, lack of information, limited physical access, economic difficulties or even discrimination. These groups, which vary from country to country, can include migrants, particularly international migrants, minority groups and slum dwellers. Programmes need to identify the groups that cannot access services and ensure that appropriate services are provided.

In the Bangladesh family planning programme, the change from a field-based to a fixed-site contraceptive delivery system is based, in part, on a desire to reduce the high cost of the family planning programme. Utilizing a fixed-site system would also allow the programme to promote more effective methods such as the IUD and sterilization. Arends-Kuenning (2002) argues, however, that fieldworkers have been most effective at meeting the family planning needs of poor and uneducated women and that removing fieldworkers completely from the family planning programme could affect the contraceptive choices that these women can make.

The issue of the extent to which national family planning programmes need to play a role in providing affordable contraceptives and other reproductive health services came forcefully to the fore during the recent "economic crisis" that affected South-East Asia and parts of East Asia. The crisis raised fears that large segments of the population might not be able to obtain contraception in those countries, such as Thailand, where increasing proportions of women had begun to access contraception through the private sector. Prachuabmoh and Mithranon (2002) report on the results of a pilot study in Thailand that indicate that although overall the crisis appeared to have little impact on the use of contraception, those women most affected by the crisis were the most likely to report that they would abort if they became pregnant. These results suggest that in a context such as that of Thailand, where low-fertility preferences have become so entrenched, contraceptives are seen as a priority good and will be purchased even in poor personal economic circumstances. The desire to avoid pregnancy in these situations, however, may also lead to higher levels of abortion when contraceptive failure occurs. In order to not place an undue burden on poor couples and provide them with affordable and effective contraception, family planning services are still required for vulnerable groups in societies where fertility has reached low levels.

Some might also argue that family planning programmes may also play a role where the policy objective of a "low-fertility" country is to increase fertility. McDonald (2002) in reviewing public policy options to increasing fertility does not mention a role for family planning programmes, although he does see an active role for policy in this area. Those countries where fertility has declined to such low levels that a policy response to increase fertility has been elicited, have primarily been developed countries where national family planning programmes have not existed. As an increasing number of developing Asian countries reach a point where increasing fertility is seen as an objective, national family planning programmes could play a role through providing fertility services for those who cannot afford to access the private sector and through promoting positive attitudes towards childbearing (see also Harbison and Robinson 2002).

Providing services to the unmarried

The second priority area identified by Jones and Leete (2002) is to ensure that the unmarried have adequate access to reproductive health information and services. Demographic and social transformations in the

Asian and Pacific region have led to calls for a greater focus on the reproductive health of adolescents. Adolescents are one of the fastest growing segments of the population. Rising ages of marriage also result in longer periods during which adolescents remain unmarried. This trend, combined with social changes that are weakening social norms against premarital sex, is resulting in higher levels of sexual activity among the unmarried (Mehta and others 1998; Gubhaju 2002).

Increased levels of sexual relations among the young, subsequent increases in levels of premarital pregnancy and the spread of sexually transmitted diseases among the young are of concern to many policy makers. Increases in levels of unsafe abortion among the unmarried (Ahman and Shah 2002) and high proportions of adolescents among those persons infected with HIV are further indications of the dire need for reproductive and sexual health services for the unmarried. It should be noted, however, that where adolescent reproductive health services are provided, in the majority of instances, activities have been confined to providing adolescents with "family values education".

The provision of adolescent reproductive health services is constrained by cultural proscriptions about providing sexual information to adolescents, particularly the unmarried, and widespread beliefs that providing information on sexual issues will lead to an increase in premarital sexual behaviour. The result is limited political commitment to establish and/or strengthen adolescent reproductive health programmes.

At a UNFPA-sponsored workshop in 2000 that reviewed the existing situation of adolescent reproductive health in East and South-East Asia and the Pacific island countries, the lack of reproductive and sexual health knowledge of adolescents was highlighted (UNFPA 2000). Many issues raised during the workshop revolved around the greater vulnerability, and the more severe consequences resulting from sexual behaviour, of adolescent girls compared with boys. For both sexes it was noted that parents generally did not discuss sexual issues with their adolescent children, that school-based programmes on sexual education were either non-existent or extremely limited in their approaches and that adolescents lacked resources to access private sector reproductive health services.

The use of public sector services is often restricted for adolescents. Many countries in the region restrict access to publicly funded family planning services to married women of reproductive age. Even in programmes where unmarried persons can theoretically use services, provider's perceptions may hinder their access. Tu and others (2002), in a study of family planning workers' attitudes to providing sexual and reproductive health services to unmarried youth in China, found that many providers expressed reservations about providing services to the unmarried. Tangmunkongvorakul and others (2002) report that providers in both the public and private sectors in northern Thailand were ambivalent about providing reproductive health services to unmarried youth, and tended to view unmarried clients in a negative light. Given the reception that they are likely to receive when seeking reproductive health services, it is not surprising that many unmarried adolescents are hesitant to seek services from the formal health sector.

The proposed "Pattaya Programme of Action on Adolescent Reproductive Health" made recommendations to improve adolescent reproductive health that were aimed at the individual, provider and societal levels (UNFPA, 2000). Concentrated efforts to change some of the underlying societal factors that increase the vulnerability of adolescents in the areas of reproductive health, particularly those factors related to gender inequality, were recommended. These efforts are required to bring about long-term change. However, the removal of barriers to providing friendly and respectful reproductive and sexual services to adolescents should be the immediate programme priority. Preventive programmes that stress abstinence from sexual relations are needed and innovative ways to present information about the benefits of abstinence to youth should be explored. Where abstinence is not possible or is not the choice made by the unmarried, reproductive health services that include the provision of affordable contraception should be made available.

Improving sexual health

In addition to and in some ways crosscutting the two areas discussed above, a further priority area for family planning programmes should be to integrate sexual health services into their services. Although sexual health is included in the definition of reproductive health of the ICPD Programme of Action, there were few recommendations on how the provision of sexual health services should be improved. In assessing how countries in the Asian and Pacific region had adjusted their reproductive health programmes after ICPD, Abdullah (1999) observed that apart from sex education for adolescents, few countries appear to have incorporated aspects of sexuality or sexual health into their programmes.

A major difficulty in attempting to incorporate sexual health into family planning and other aspects of reproductive health is the sensitivity associated with discussing topics related to sex. Even researchers have tended to shy away from directly researching aspects of sexuality. Hawkes, Pachauri and Mane (2002) note information on sexuality in Asia has been limited until recently and it has only been the impact of HIV/AIDS that has spurred efforts to understand more deeply the relationship between sexual and reproductive health.

Dixon-Mueller (1993) argues that family planning providers need to learn about the sexual preferences of their clients in order to provide services that meet their clients' particular needs. For example, the type of contraceptive preferred may relate to how it affects sexual relationships. In providing STI services, it is also important to understand the sexual practices of clients. However, except for NGOs, there have been only sporadic attempts to provide family planning workers with counselling skills in the area of sexuality.

The issue of gender-based power imbalances in sexual relationships is of particular salience for reproductive health. Lack of power takes away the ability to make choices. Where this lack of choice occurs in the context of sexual relations, it can lead to adverse reproductive health outcomes. Such outcomes can include the inability to protect oneself against STIs or unwanted pregnancy, being denied access to reproductive health services or being denied sexual pleasure (see Blanc 2001).

Blanc (2001, p. 208) calls for programme interventions that attempt to ameliorate power imbalances in relationships as a strategy for improving aspects of reproductive health. She notes that improving spousal communication seems to be important "in preventive behavior for HIV/AIDS and STIs as well as in the prevention of unwanted pregnancies and the improvement of sexual pleasure". A study of married couples in India also found that there was very limited communication among spouses about RTIs and that this lack of communication affected treatment-seeking behaviour (Santhya and Dasvarma 2002).

There is increasing evidence of high levels of non-consensual sex, particularly among adolescents. Gubhaju (2002), in reviewing some of the limited research available on this topic for Asia, notes many young women in relationships are at particular risk of being coerced into sex. Such coercion can also occur in work situations where males have authority over women. Evidence from a study in rural India indicated that a high proportion of abortions among unmarried women resulted from decisions to end unwanted pregnancies that were outcomes of non-consensual sex (Ganatra and Hirve 2002). We have little information in Asia about the males being coerced into sex.

The whole issue of gender-based violence has received scant programme attention and little research attention in Asia. Hardee and others (1999, p. s8) in their review of the post-Cairo progress of eight countries, including Bangladesh, India and Nepal, concluded that "gender-based violence remains outside the scope of most programs".

Family planning in reproductive health programmes

Family planning programmes have several well-documented advantages in providing broader reproductive health services. This includes the presence of a network that in many countries reaches down to the village level. Through this network it is possible to disseminate information and provide basic services to the bulk of the population. Family planning workers are also well versed in dealing with sensitive topics. In many societies, family planning has been considered to be a private matter and it has taken considerable time and effort to enable family planning workers to discuss contraceptive issues. In areas such as the provision of HIV/AIDS services, family planning workers would seem to have an initial advantage in taking on this role. The basis for this new role is that AIDS is primarily a sexually transmitted disease. In the provision of contraceptive services, family planning personnel have shown that it is possible to discuss matters that are sexually related, although much more training is required in this area. Finally, the condom is well known in many countries as a contraceptive method and its use as a dual-protection method could be promoted within this context.

In order to take full advantage of family planning programmes in providing other reproductive health services, there is, however, a need to expand the perceptions of the target populations of clients. Family planning programmes in most countries have been established to target married women of reproductive age. As noted above, this often means that interests of other segments of the population, such as unmarried women, are often ignored. The focus on married women of reproductive age can also result in negative outcomes for this target population. For example, one of the most effective strategies for treating RTIs, including STIs, for women in low resource settings is using the syndromic approach to manage male urethral discharge and genital ulcers. Treatment of males is very effective in reducing transmission of infection to their female partners. Applying the syndromic approach to women is less effective because of the large proportion of women who are asymptomatic, or who may be reinfected by their male partners after their own treatment (Haberland and others 2002). Given the more limited power that women have in influencing the conditions of sexual relations, prevention activities directed at women will be less effective unless their male partners are also included. As family planning programmes evolve into more comprehensive reproductive health programmes, they must actively seek to involve both women and men in their programmes.

In the regional review of progress towards integration of reproductive health services, Walker (1998) concluded that significant progress had been made in integrating services. He notes that further progress requires a better understanding of how gender issues influence the provision and use of reproductive health services. The need to clearly define what services are to be integrated and the resource needs for such integration are also cited as necessary practical elements in taking integration forward. These issues remain central to efforts to integrate family planning with other reproductive health services.

Conclusion

During and following ICPD, concern was expressed that the emphasis on reproductive rights of women would weaken family planning efforts. This concern was rooted in the view that family planning programmes were a key factor in constraining fertility and that reducing the primacy accorded to family planning programmes within the area of reproductive health would be detrimental to long-held societal goals of reducing birth rates. This view is still held by many.

However, the experience accumulated in the eight years since ICPD should help to allay these fears. The integration of family planning into expanded reproductive health programmes that provide women and men with choice in planning their reproductive lives, while still incomplete, has not led to reversals in fertility decline. Couples in very diverse contexts throughout the region have demonstrated that they wish to choose the number of children they have and under what conditions they have those children. At the individual level, this may mean a need for reproductive health services to provide assistance to couples that cannot reach their desired family size. But for the majority of couples it means providing them with choice to limit their fertility while enjoying a healthy life.

What is required is efforts to systematically document and disseminate the efforts that have been made to change the reproductive health services to become more responsive to clients. Through exposure to the successful impacts of changes in policies and programmes, decision makers may be more likely to support the fundamental changes required to implement a reproductive rights- based approach to reproductive health. At the same time, there needs to be continuing research, particularly in the form of evaluation of pilot projects, to address some of the issues that are of concern to policy makers.

The issues from the Programme of Action where considerable work remains to be undertaken are many. Some of the priority areas are related to difficulties in transforming cultural values that support an environment and that limit the informed choice of individuals belonging to some groups in the population. For example, the development of adolescent reproductive health programmes has been hampered by the widespread belief that unmarried adolescents should not be exposed to information and/or services related to reproductive health. Entrenched systems that support gender inequality also restrict choices available to women while some societies provide legitimation for limited involvement of men in reproductive health.

There is also the need to move forward from considering only ICPD in considering how to improve reproductive health. As noted in this paper, the interrelationships between sexual relationships and reproductive health were not a main focus at ICPD. However, the centrality of sexual relationships to reproductive health cannot be disputed and there is an urgent need for programme interventions aimed at fostering reproductive health through improving the quality of sexual relationships for both men and women. Family planning programmes, while not the only institutions that can be utilized to improve sexual health, are ideally placed to provide such services.

Family planning programmes remain central to reproductive health. In many countries of the region, some of the more traditional roles of family planning programmes, such as the provision of free contraception and efforts made to change family size norms, are of declining programme relevance. In other countries, these activities remain important. In all programmes as one moves forward efforts to foster improvements in reproductive health in the region, further development of family planning services within the context of improving the sexual and reproductive choices of women and men is required. Family planning programmes must ensure that the poor and other vulnerable groups are able to access quality family planning and other reproductive health services.

References

Abdullah, Rashidah (1999). "Overview", in *Taking up the Cairo Challenge* (Kuala Lumpur, Asian-Pacific Resource and Research Centre for Women.), pp. 3-16.

Ahman, Elisabeth and Iqbal Shah (2002). "Unsafe abortion: worldwide estimates for 2000", *Reproductive Health Matters,* vol. 10, No. 19, pp. 13-17.

Arends-Kuenning, Mary (2002). "Reconsidering the doorstep-delivery system in the Bangladesh family planning program", *Studies in Family Planning,* vol. 33, No. 1, pp. 87-102.

Attané, Isabelle (2002). "China's family planning policy: an overview of its past and future", *Studies in Family Planning,* vol. 33, No. 1, pp. 103-113.

Bairagi, Radheshyam (2001). "Effects of sex preference on contraceptive use, abortion and fertility in Matlab, Bangladesh", *International Family Planning Perspectives,* vol. 27, No. 3, pp. 137-143.

Bang, Rani and others (1989) "High prevalence of gynaecological diseases in rural Indian women", *The Lancet,* January, pp. 85-88.

Berer, Marge and T.K. Sundari Ravindran (1999). "Preventing maternal mortality: evidence, resources, leadership, action", in Marge Berer and T.K. Sundari Ravindran, eds., *Safe Motherhood Initiatives: Critical Issues* (Oxford, Blackwell Science).

Bhatia, Jagdish and John Cleland (1995). "Self-reported symptoms of gynecological morbidity and their treatment in South India", *Studies in Family Planning*, vol. 26, No. 4, pp. 203-216.

Blanc, Ann (2001). "The effect of power in sexual relationships on sexual and reproductive health", *Studies in Family Planning, vol. 32, No. 3, pp. 189-213.*

Bruce, Judith (1990). "Fundamental elements of the quality of care: a simple framework", *Studies in Family Planning*, vol. 21, No. 2, pp. 61-91.

Caldwell, John, James Phillips and Barkat-e-Khuda (2002). "The future of family planning programs", *Studies in Family Planning,* vol. 33, No. 1, pp. 1-10.

Dixon-Mueller, Ruth (1993). *Population Policy and Women's Rights: Transforming Reproductive Choice* (New York, Praeger).

East West Center (2002). *The Future of Population in Asia* (Honolulu, East-West Center).

ESCAP (1998). *Asia-Pacific Population Policies and Programmes: Future Directions*, Asian Population Studies Series No. 153 (United Nations publication, Sales No. E.99.II.F.4).

Fortney, Judith (1987). "The importance of family planning in reducing maternal mortality", *Studies in Family Planning*, vol. 18, No. 2, pp. 109-114.

Ganatra, Bela and Siddhi Hirve (2002). "Induced abortions among adolescent women in rural Maharashtra", *Reproductive Health Matters*, vol. 10, No. 19, pp. 76-85.

Greenspan, Allison (1993). "Changes in fertility patterns can improve child survival in Southeast Asia", Asia-Pacific Population and Policy Paper No. 27 (Honolulu, East-West Center).

Gu, Baochang, Ruth Simmons and Diana Szatkowski (2002). "Offering a choice of contraceptive methods in Deqing county, China: changing practice in the family planning program since 1995", in Nicole Haberland and Diana Measham, eds., *Responding to Cairo* (New York Population Council), pp. 58-73.

Gubhaju, Bhakta (2002). "Adolescent reproductive health in Asia", paper presented at the IUSSP Conference on Southeast Asia's Population in a Changing Asian Context, Bangkok, 10-13 June.

Haberland, Nicole and others (2002). "Pitfalls and possibilities: managing RTIs in the family planning and general reproductive health services", in Nicole Haberland and Diana Measham, eds., *Responding to Cairo* (New York, Population Council), pp. 99-113.

Harbison, Sarah and Warren Robinson (2002). "Policy implications of the next world demographic transition", *Studies in Family Planning*, vol. 33, No. 1, pp. 37-48.

Hardee, Karen and others (1999). "Reproductive health policies and programs in eight countries: progress since Cairo", *International Family Planning Perspectives*, vol. 25 (Supplement), pp. S2-S9.

Hawkes, Sarah, Saroj Pachauri and Purnima Mane (2002). "Editorial introduction", *Culture, Health & Sexuality*, vol. 4, No. 2, pp. 125-131.

Hull, Terrence (1998). "The challenge of contraceptive implant removals in East Nusa Tenggara, Indonesia", *International Family Planning Perspectives*, vol. 24, No. 4, pp. 176-179.

Institute for Health Sciences (IHS) (2002). "Reproductive health and reproductive health services in rural China and Yunnan", unpublished paper (Kunming Medical College).

Jain, Anrudh and others (2002). "Learning about clients' needs: family planning field workers in the Philippines", in Nicole Haberland and Diana Measham, eds., *Responding to Cairo* (New York, Population Council) pp. 99-113.

Johansson, Annika and others (1996). "Abortion in context: women's experience in two villages in Thai Binh province, Vietnam", *International Family Planning Perspectives*, vol. 22, No. 3, pp. 103-107.

Jones, Gavin (1998). "The Bali Declaration and the Programme of Action of the International Conference on Population and Development in the context of the population dynamics of the Asian and Pacific region", in ESCAP, *Asia-Pacific Population Policies and Programmes: Future Directions*, Asian Population Studies Series No. 153 (United Nations publication, Sales No. E.99.II.F.4), pp. 59-78.

___________ and Richard Leete (2002). "Asia's family planning programmes as low fertility is attained", *Studies in Family Planning*, vol. 33, No. 1 , pp. 114-126.

Kaufman, Joan and others (1999). "A study of field-based methods for diagnosing reproductive tract infections in rural Yunnan Province, China", *Studies in Family Planning*, vol. 30, No. 2, pp. 112-119.

Khan, Atiqur Rahman, Tan Boon-Ann and Suman Mehta (1998). "Quality of care and target-free approach for family planning programmes", in ESCAP, *Asia-Pacific Population Policies and Programmes: Future Directions*, Asian Population Studies Series No. 153 (United Nations publication, Sales No. E.99.II.F.4), pp. 145-166.

Knodel, John,. Aphichat Chamratrithirong and Nibhon Debavalya (1987). *Thailand's Reproductive Revolution* (Madison, University of Wisconsin Press).

Koenig, Michael, Gillian Foo and Ketan Joshi (2000). "Quality of care within the Indian family welfare programme: a review of recent evidence", *Studies in Family Planning*, vol. 31, No. 1, pp. 1-18.

Lien Phan Thi and others (2002). "The prevalence of reproductive tract infection in Hue, Vietnam", *Studies in Family Planning*, vol. 33, No. 3, pp. 217-226.

Luther, N.Y., S. Thapa and S.B. Westley, (1999). "Nepal survey shows that 'family planning saves lives'", Asia-Pacific Population and Policy Paper No. 29 (Honolulu, East-West Center).

McDonald, Peter (2002). "Sustaining fertility through public policy", *Population*, vol. 57, No. 3, pp. 417-446.

Mehta, Suman, Riet Groenen and Francisco Roque (1998). "Adolescents in changing times: Issues and perspectives for adolescent reproductive health in the ESCAP region", in ESCAP, *Asia-Pacific Population Policies and Programmes: Future Directions*, Asian Population Studies Series No. 153 (United Nations publication, Sales No. E.99.II.F.4), pp. 167-194.

Miller, Jane and others (1992). "Birth spacing and child mortality in Bangladesh and the Philippines", *Demography*, vol. 29, No. 2, pp. 305-318.

Murthy, Nirmala and others (2002). "Dismantling India's contraceptive target system: and overview and three case studies", in Nicole Haberland and Diana Measham, eds., *Responding to Cairo* (New York, Population Council), pp. 25-57.

Popkin, Barry and others (1993). "Nutrition, lactation and birth spacing in Filipino women", *Demography*, vol. 30, No. 3, pp. 333-352.

Potts, Malcolm and others (1999). "Paying for reproductive health care: what is needed and what is available?", *International Family Planning Perspectives*, vol. 25 (Supplement), pp. S10-S16.

Prachuabmoh, Vipan and Preeya Mithranon (2002). "Below-replacement fertility in Thailand and its policy implications", paper prepared for the Workshop on Fertility Decline, Below Replacement Fertility and the Family in Asia: Prospects, Consequences and Policies, National University of Singapore, 10-12 April.

Ross, John and others (2002). "Contraceptive method choice in developing countries", *International Family Planning Perspectives*, vol. 28, No. 1, pp. 32-40.

Santhya, K.G. and Gour Dasvarma (2002). "Spousal communication on reproductive illness among rural women in southern India", *Culture, Health & Sexuality*, vol. 4, No. 2, pp. 223-236.

Schuler, Sidney Ruth and Zakir Hossain (1998). "Family planning clinics through women's eyes and voices: a case study from rural Bangladesh", *International Family Planning Perspectives*, vol. 24, No. 4, pp. 170-175.

Tangmunkongvorakul, Anurat and others (2002). "Providers' perspectives in addressing sexual and reproductive health needs in northern Thailand", paper presented at the IUSSP Conference on Southeast Asia's Population in a Changing Asian Context, Bangkok, 10-13 June.

Tu, Xiaowen, Nian Cui and Ersheng Gao (2002). "Attitudes of family planning workers on the provision of sexual and reproductive health services to unmarried young adults in China", paper presented at the IUSSP Conference on Southeast Asia's Population in a Changing Asian Context, Bangkok, 10-13 June.

UNFPA (2000). "Report of the UNFPA Intercountry Workshop Adolescent Reproductive Health for East and South-East Asia and the Pacific Island Countries" (Bangkok, UNFPA).

Walker, Godfrey (1998). "Implementation challenges of reproductive health, including family planning and sexual health: issues concerning the integration of reproductive health components", in ESCAP, *Asia-Pacific Population Policies and Programmes: Future Directions*, Asian Population Studies Series No. 153 (United Nations publication, Sales No. E.99.II.F.4), pp. 115-144.

Winckler, Edwin (2002). "Chinese reproductive policy at the turn of the millennium: dynamic stability", *Population and Development Review*, vol. 28, No. 3, pp. 379-418.

WHO (1998). *Unsafe Abortion: Global and Regional Estimates of Incidence of a Mortality due to Unsafe Abortion.* (Geneva, WHO).

Asia-Pacific Population Journal Guidelines for Contributors

The quarterly *Asia-Pacific Population Journal* is a periodical produced by the Emerging Social Issues Division of the United Nations Economic and Social Commission for Asia and the Pacific (ESCAP), with support from ESCAP and the United Nations Population Fund (UNFPA). Its purpose is to provide a medium for the international exchange of knowledge, experience, ideas, technical information and data on all aspects of the field of population in order to assist developing countries in the region in improving the utilization of data and information for policy and programme purposes, among others.

Original contributions are invited, especially papers by authors from or familiar with the Asian and Pacific region. Ideally those papers will discuss the policy and/or programme implications of population issues and solutions to problems and will report on experiences from which others may benefit.

Note to contributors

All material submitted for the consideration of the Editorial Board should be in the English language. The paper, prepared in one of the major word-processing programs, should be supplied in "hard-copy" form with a diskette (3 ½ inch) or sent by e-mail attachment to the address indicated below. Ideally, the printed copy will be typewritten in double spacing on one side only of white A4 paper. The margins should be generous, at least 3 cm (roughly 1 inch) wide, preferably more for the left-hand margin. The paper should be within approximately 7,000 words including tables, figures, references, etc. It should include a short abstract (100-200 words) of the issues addressed and the most important findings.

A complete list of references arranged alphabetically by author should also be included at the end of the manuscript. Please refer to examples in any issue of the *Journal*. Figures and tables should be supplied on diskette, preferably in any major spread sheet program or in Microsoft Excel.

Manuscripts are accepted on the understanding that they are subject to editorial revision. Contributors should indicate in an accompanying statement or letter that the material has not previously been published or submitted for publication elsewhere.

A brief introduction about the author(s) (title and affiliations, and so forth) should also be included.

As all manuscripts will be subject to peer review by professionals in the field, the name(s) of the author(s) or other identifying information should be placed on the title page only in order to preserve anonymity. Manuscripts may be sent by airmail or e-mail to the Editor, Emerging Social Issues Division, ESCAP, United Nations Building, Rajdamnern Nok Avenue, Bangkok 10200, Thailand, e-mail: escap-population@un.org